Radiology of Influenza

Hongjun Li
Editor

Radiology of Influenza

A Practical Approach

Springer

Editor
Hongjun Li
Capital Medical University
Beijing You An Hospital
Beijing
China

ISBN 978-94-024-0906-2 ISBN 978-94-024-0908-6 (eBook)
DOI 10.1007/978-94-024-0908-6

Library of Congress Control Number: 2016954030

Printed on acid-free paper

This Springer imprint is published by Springer Nature
The registered company is Springer Science+Business Media B.V. Dordrecht

Foreword

Radiological study of influenza targets on the diseases caused by influenza virus and its subtypes to characterize the radiological signs of lesions and their evolution based on clinical staging and pathological findings.

Although influenza is a common disease, it is characterized by global transmission, repeated occurrence all year round, high incidence, wide involvement, and great harm to human health, which should attract scholarly attention. It is necessary to set up special research projects for systematic study to reveal the characteristic radiological signs and to assess its application value in clinical practice. Systemic studies can also enrich and extend the theory of medical radiology and contribute to improving clinical management of pneumonia induced by influenza. Previously, human infected avian influenza was caused by subtypes H1N1, H1N2, and H3N2 of type A influenza virus. And subtypes of avian influenza virus have shown their capability to cross the species barrier and infect human. On February 19, 2013, the first case of human infected H7N9 avian influenza was reported in Shanghai, China. In May 9, 2013, WHO announced that 131 cases with definitive laboratory diagnosis were reported, including 32 cases of death. By June 30, 2013, a total of 134 cases were definitively diagnosed, including 43 cases of death. In the subsequent period of time, sporadic cases of human infected H7N9 avian influenza were reported in different areas of China. The clinical manifestations of human infected avian influenza vary from asymptomatic infection and mild upper respiratory tract symptoms to severe pneumonia and multiple organs failure. Because radiological findings are the demonstrations of pathological changes and the pathological changes are the basis of radiological signs, radiology plays important roles in monitoring the changes of lesions, non-invasive diagnosis, and therapeutic assessment. Along with the rapid social and economic development and the changes of human life style, influenza control is no longer a national or regional issue, but a global issue. The disciplinary construction should be focused on global strategic top-level design. Only a global holistic strategy can effectively prevent and control influenza, and thus guarantee the human well being and national security. From these perspectives, we systematically summarized radiological signs of each clinical type of influenza to gain more knowledge about influenza. In such a way, we intended to extend our understanding about the occurrence, development, and evolution of influenza, which help in formulating appropriate therapeutic plan. In addition, we chose a format of case guidance to facilitate reading, understanding, and clinical use.

This book is characterized by systemic introduction of the epidemiology, clinical symptoms, pathomechanism, laboratory tests, and radiological findings of each type of influenza. This book has rich contents, complete images and data, and typical cases demonstration, which can be satisfactorily used in research, clinical practice, and pedagogy.

The data and radiological images in this book were from many hospitals in China. Their contributions help this book to come into being. Here, on behalf of the editorial committee of this book, I would like to express my sincere gratitude to the commitment, obligation, and sincerity from the collaborative hospitals!

The editing of this book was supported and assisted by LI Ning, the president of Beijing Youan Hospital (Affiliated to Capital Medical University, Beijing, China), and my team members, to whom I expresses my heartfelt thanks here!

The editing of this book was invited and funded by Science Press, Beijing, and we express our gratitude to the leaders and editors in publication of this book!

We hope that the publication of this book will play a role in inducing more publications in this research area. And we also sincerely hope that it obtain understanding and help from colleagues in radiology. The development of a discipline is a process of gradual understanding and advancing. And the weaknesses are unavoidable and need to be improved. We expect our colleagues in radiology point out the weaknesses so as to improve this book.

The editing of this book was supported by Specific Foundation for Development of Clinical Medicine by Beijing Municipal Hospital Authority (Project No. ZYLX201511).

Beijing, China Hongjun Li

Brief Introduction

Influenza is an acute respiratory tract disease caused by influenza virus, with high infectivity and rapid transmission. The research team, led by Prof. LI Hongjun, for the first time systematically summarized the disease spectrum of influenza based on careful screening of the typical cases and their studies from perspectives of clinical data, radiological data, autopsy, and pathological contrasts. Such a systemic study was to systematically reveal the radiological evolution of the lesions as well as their underlying pathological mechanisms. Therefore, such a systematic study provides valuable, scientific, and rigorous first-hand information for the diagnosis, prevention, treatment, and scientific research of influenza and its complications.

This book, instead of just plain text, integrated literature review and case study, which helps the readers to obtain more comprehensive knowledge from both theoretical and practical perspectives. Therefore, a compound structure was selected that is more readers friendly than singular atlas, literature review, or title introduction. The whole book is composed of 2 parts including 13 chapters. The first part is the general introduction, which mainly elucidates the basic theories about etiology, epidemiology, and radiological examinations of influenza. The second part introduces various types of influenza, specifically including influenza, type A H1N1 influenza, human infected H5N1 avian influenza, human infected H7N9 avian influenza, human infected H5N6 avian influenza, and human infected H10N8 avian influenza. Each chapter is focused on one disease with several typical cases, which were elucidated with complete case history, laboratory tests findings, pathological figures, and radiological data (X-ray and CT scan). And each clinical case is characterized by the completeness of the clinical data, typical radiological images, and detailed key points for differential diagnosis. The discussion section in the case study clinches the point and helps the clinicians to differentiate similar radiological signs and thus make accurate diagnosis. This book is recommendable to clinicians working in the department of diagnostic imaging and other clinical departments as well as students studying medicine.

Editorial Committee Members

Honorary Editors: Ning Li, Shiyuan Liu

Editors: Hongjun Li

Associate Editors: Puxuan Lu, Yuxin Shi, Bailu Liu, Hongzhou Lu, Li Li, Lu Wang, Liyi Wang

Editorial Committee Members (in alphabetic order):

Qi An Shenzhen Third People's Hospital, Affiliated to Guangdong Medical College, Shenzhen, Guangdong, China

Dongwu Bao Nanyang Medical College, Nanyang, Henan, China

Dongying Bao Beijing Youan Hospital, Affiliated to Capital Medical University, Beijing, China

Jie Dai Department of Pathology, Capital Medical University, Beijing, China

Qunyi Deng Shenzhen Third People's Hospital, Affiliated to Guangdong Medical College, Shenzhen, Guangdong, China

Xiang Gao Nanchang First People's Hospital, Nanchang, Jiangxi, China

Yang Ge Fuyang Second People's Hospital, Fuyang, Anhui, China

Yinglin Guo Taiping People's Hospital, Daowai District, Harbin, Heilongjiang, China

Jian He Nanchang First People's Hospital, Nanchang, Jiangxi, China

Su Hu Affiliated First Hospital, Suzhou University, Suzhou, Jiangsu, China

Chunhong Hu Affiliated First Hospital, Suzhou University, Suzhou, Jiangsu, China

Yanan Hu Guangzhou University of Chinese Medicine, Guangzhou, Guangdong, China

Lili Jiang Linyl People's Hospital, Linyi, Shandong, China

Haiying Jin Affiliated Huaihe Hospital, Henan University, Kaifeng, Henan, China

Lili Kong Yeda Hospital, Yantai, Shandong, China

Qun Lao Hangzhou Children's Hospital, Hangzhou, Zhejiang, China

Li Li Beijing Youan Hospital, Capital Medical University, Beijing, China

Min Li Suzhou Fifth People's Hospital, Suzhou, Jiangsu, China

Ping Li Affiliated Second Hospital, Harbin Medical University, Harbin, Heilongjiang, China

Hongchen Li Health Care Center, Baihe Town, Yuancheng District, Nanyang, Henan, China

Hongchi Li Center for Family Planning, Wolong District, Nanyang, Henan, China

Hongjun Li Beijing Youan Hospital, Capital Medical University, Beijing, China

Hongyan Li Affiliated First Hospital, Nanyang Medical College, Nanyang, Henan, China

Jingjing Li Affiliated Shenzhen Third People's Hospital, Guangdong Medical College, Shenzhen, Guangdong, China

Xueqin Li Beijing Youan Hospital, Capital Medical University, Beijing, China

Jiafu Lin Affiliated Hospital, Chuanbei Medical College, Nanchong, Sichuan, China

Bailu Liu Affiliated Second Hospital, Harbin Medical University, Harbin, Heilongjiang, China

Wenya Liu Affiliated First Hospital, Xinjiang Medical University, Urumuqi, Xinjiang, China

Yingxia Liu Affiliated Shenzhen Third People's Hospital, Guangdong Medical College, Shenzhen, Guangdong, China

Hongzhou Lu Affiliated Clinical Center of Public Health, Fudan University, Shanghai, China

Puxuan Lu Affiliated Shenzhen Third People's Hospital, Guangdong Medical College, Shenzhen, Guangdong, China

Shengxiu Lv Chongqing Medical Rescuing Center of Public Health, Chongqing, China

Wei Ma Affiliated Shenzhen Third People's Hospital, Guangdong Medical College, Shenzhen, Guangdong, China

Xiangui Ran Fuyang Second People's Hospital, Fuyang, Anhui, China

Meiji Ren Beijing Youan Hospital, Capital Medical University, Beijing, China

Yuxin Shi Affiliated Clinical Center of Public Health, Fudan University, Shanghai, China

Fengxiang Song Affiliated Clinical Center of Public Health, Fudan University, Shanghai, China

Li Sun Mudanjiang Second People's Hospital, Mudanjiang, Heilongjiang, China

Hong Wang Affiliated Second Hospital, Xinjiang Medical University, Urumuqi, Xinjiang, China

Jian Wang Affiliated First Hospital, Xinjiang Medical University, Urumuqi, Xinjiang, China

Lu Wang Zhangzhongjing Hospital of Chinese Medicine, Nanyang, Henan, China

Guixia Wang Affiliated Hospital, Chuanbei Medical College, Nanchong, Sichuan, China

Guokun Wang Affiliated Second Hospital, Harbin Medical University, Harbin, Heilongjiang, China

Haopeng Wang Affiliated Shenzhen Third People's Hospital, Guangdong Medical College, Shenzhen, Guangdong, China

Liyi Wang Affiliated First Hospital, Nanyang Medical College, Nanyang, Henan, China

Xiaohong Wang Huaihe Hospital, Henan University, Kaifeng, Henan, China

Zipeng Wang Affiliated Second Hospital, Harbin Medical University, Harbin, Heilongjiang, China

Guilin Yang Affiliated Shenzhen Third People's Hospital, Guangdong Medical College, Shenzhen, Guangdong, China

Xuhua Yang Kangan Hospital, Mudanjiang, Heilongjiang, China

Yuxin Yang Xinjiang Sixth People's Hospital, Urumuqi, Xinjiang, China

Weiye Yu Affiliated Shenzhen Third People's Hospital, Guangdong Medical College, Shenzhen, Guangdong, China

Hong Yuan Affiliated Shenzhen Third People's Hospital, Guangdong Medical College, Shenzhen, Guangdong, China

Jing Yuan Affiliated Shenzhen Third People's Hospital, Guangdong Medical College, Shenzhen, Guangdong, China

Shaohua Zhai Qu Affiliated Hospital, Chuanbei Medical College, Nanchong, Sichuan, China

Yue Zeng Affiliated Hospital, Chuanbei Medical College, Nanchong, Sichuan, China

Zheng Zeng Affiliated Shenzhen Third People's Hospital, Guangdong Medical College, Shenzhen, Guangdong, China

Qingsi Zeng Affiliated First Hospital, Guangzhou Medical University, Guangzhou, Guangdong, China

Na Zhang Chengdu Clinical Center of Public Health, Chengdu, Sichuan, China

Lihong Zhang Dengzhou People's Hospital, Dengzhou, Henan, China

Qianqian Zhang Affiliated Shenzhen Third People's Hospital, Guangdong Medical College, Shenzhen, Guangdong, China

Xiaochun Zhang Affiliated First Hospital (Xinan Hospital), Third Military Medical University, Chongqing, China

Zhijun Zhang Xinjiang Sixth People's Hospital, Urumuqi, Xinjiang, China

Zhiyong Zhang Affiliated Clinical Center of Public Health, Fudan University, Shanghai, China

Dawei Zhao Beijing Youan Hospital, Capital Medical University, Beijing, China

Qingxia Zhao Zhengzhou Sixth People's Hospital, Zhengzhou, Henan, China

Boping Zhou Affiliated Shenzhen Third People's Hospital, Guangdong Medical College, Shenzhen, Guangdong, China

Jianbing Zhu Suzhou Science and Technology Town Hospital, Suzhou, Jiangsu, China

Xinping Zhu Capital Medical University

Jin Xu School of Foreign Languages, Southern Medical University, Guangzhou, China

Academic Consultants (In Alphabetic Order)

Min Chen, Jingliang Cheng, Xiaoyuan Feng, Youmin Guo, Ping Han,
Wenxiao Jia, Weijian Jiang, Zhengyu Jin, Kuncheng Li, Changhong Liang,
Guangming Lu, Baozhong Shen, Bin Song, Gaojun Teng, Peijun Wang,
Zhenchang Wang, Ke Xu, Chunshui Yu, Huishu Yuan, Mengsu Zeng,
Hui Zhang, Chunwu Zhou

Brief Introduction to the Editor

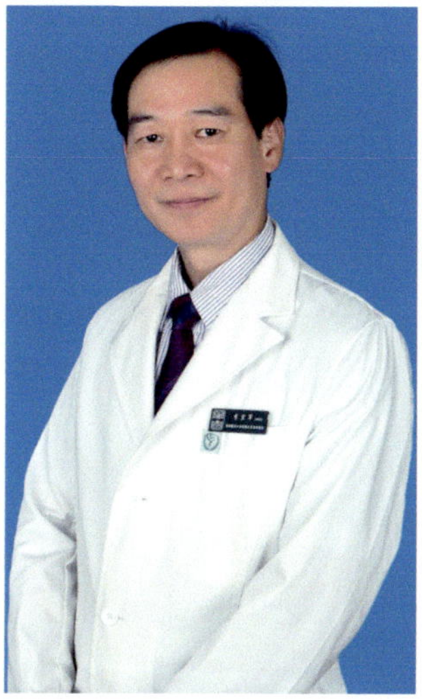

Hongjun LI, male, aged 49 years, MD, chief physician, professor, supervisor of master degree candidates in Capital Medical University and Wuhan University, overseas talent from UK, an expert receiving special allowance of the State Council due to his outstanding contribution.

Research direction: Radiology of infections and infectious diseases.

Current position: Director at Radiology Department, Affiliated Beijing Youan Hospital, Capital Medical University, Beijing, China; Deputy director at Department of Medical Imaging and Nuclear Medicine, Capital Medical University, Beijing, China; Chief-editor of Radiology of Infectious Diseases.

Social service: Expert Reviewing Committee member for Chinese Award in Medicine; Expert Reviewing Committee member for National Overseas Study Foundation, China; Reviewing Committee member for Beijing Municipal Natural Science Foundation; Chairman, Radiology committee on infectious and inflammatory diseases, Chinese research-oriented hospital; Chair of Radiology of Infection Sub-branch, Radiology Branch, Chinese Medical Association; Chair of Radiology of Infection Branch, Working and Treating Committee of Chinese HIV/AIDS and STD Association; Chair of Radiology of Infectious Diseases Management Sub-branch, Infectious Diseases Management Branch, Hospital Management Association in China; member at Abdominal Radiology Sub-branch, Radiology Branch, Chinese Medical Association; standing member at Beijing Medical Radiology Association, Chinese Medical Association; member of Korean Radiology Society; editorial committee member of 14 journals including Chinese Medical Journal.

Clinical work: Prof. LI specializes in radiological diagnosis and differential diagnosis for liver disease, infections, infectious diseases, (such as HIV/AIDS-related diseases) and is a senior radiologist specializing in radiological grading, localizing, quantitative and qualitative diagnosis of HBV-related hepatocellular carcinoma and AIDS based on clinical and pathological staging as well as noninvasive multimodal radiological biomarker.

Scientific research: Prof. LI has directed and participated in 8 national and provincial research projects and international collaborative research projects, with a total foundation of up to 10 million RMB yuan. He has published 116 papers, including 45 SCI-indexed papers (IF ranging from 1.016 to 9.416); and his research projects have been successively funded by National Natural Science Foundation, Beijing Natural Science Foundation, Beijing Sailing Program, International Publishing Fund, and Research Foundation by Ministry of Health in China for 27 times. He also have edited and published 19 books, including 6 books internationally published by Springer, and 2 books nationally published as the national blueprints. In addition, he has won 7 provincial awards including Second Prize of Chinese Science and Technology Award in Medicine as the director and holds 16 national patents and intellectual property rights as the director and/or owner.

Preface

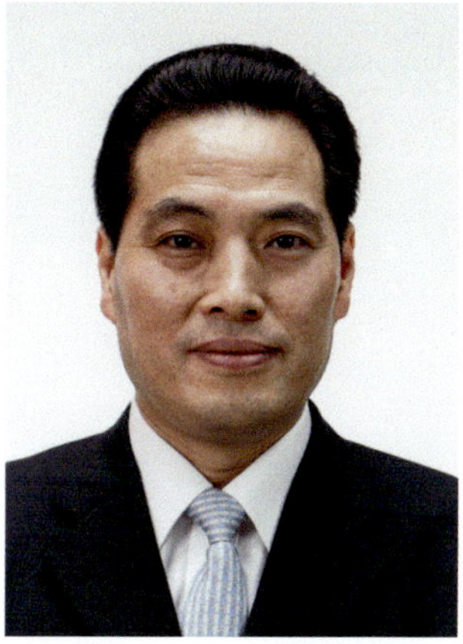

Influenza (abbreviated as flu) is an acute respiratory infectious disease caused by influenza virus, which is characterized by acute onset, rapid spread, wide prevalence, and liabilities of regional epidemic or pandemic. In various types of influenza virus, type A influenza virus often causes epidemic outbreaks and even pandemic of influenza, and small-scale epidemic of influenza occurs every 2 to 3 years. In March 2009, outbreak of human infected swine influenza occurred in Mexico, which then rapidly spread worldwide and was later nominated by WHO as type A H1N1 influenza. In May 1997, outbreak of human infected H5N1 avian influenza occurred in Hong Kong, which was the first time that human has been infected by avian influenza with consequent occurrence of death and attracted global concern. In April 2013, the first case of human infected H7N9 avian influenza was reported in eastern China, which is fatal with a high mortality rate, and its death rate in 2013 was 32.6 %. Following the cases of human infected H7N9 avian influenza, the cases of human infected H5N6 and H10N8 avian influenza were reported. The outbreaks and epidemics of influenza negatively affect human health and the quality of life, and consume a large quantity of health care resources that result in substantial loss both socially and economically.

Complication is the main cause of death in patients with influenza; therefore, the early diagnosis and differential diagnosis of complications constitute the key factor influencing the survival rate and life quality in patients with influenza. Radiological examination is an important procedure for the diagnosis and differential diagnosis of complications. Targeting on the plain facts about influenza and its complications, Prof. LI collaborated with radiologists from dozens of hospitals in China to integrate multi-center resources and analyzed the data of patients with influenza systematically and comprehensively. With their collective efforts, this book, *Radiology of Influenza*, has been edited. This book, based on typical clinical cases, elucidated the etiology, pathology, clinical manifestation, radiological finding, and differential diagnosis of various complications following influenza. A discussion section at the final part of each case study puts forward comments and clinical experience to elucidate radiological findings of each complication following influenza. Such a well-structured format is intended to provide more practical guidance and reference for radiologists and clinicians.

This book covers 2 parts including 13 chapters in about 0.2 million words with more than 300 figures. The text and figures are in a well-structured format to demonstrate the main radiological signs of influenza for convenience of reading. And this book provides a favorable reference for the diagnosis and therapeutic assessment of influenza.

Deputy Director of Radiology Branch, Chinese Medical Association Shiyuan Liu

Contents

Part I

Basic Theory About Influenza

Overview of Influenza

1

Jian Wang

1.1 Definition

Influenza, abbreviated as flu, is an acute respiratory tract infection caused by influenza virus. And it is characterized by strong infectivity and rapid transmission.

Radiological studies on influenza concern description and evolution of lesions caused by invasion of influenza virus and its subtypes, which are based on the clinical staging of influenza and the respective pathological features.

1.2 Clinical Manifestation

After infection of influenza virus, the patients typically experience acute onset of high fever, systemic soreness, significant fatigue and mild respiratory symptoms. Acute onset of high fever is the most typical symptom of influenza and also the initial symptom of influenza. The patients usually sustain high fever that persists for 3–5 days, with a body temperature of up to 39–40 °C. Influenza is highly prevalent during autumns and winters whose occurrence aggravates many potentially existing diseases, such as heart and/or lung diseases, and may be further complicated by pneumonia, bronchitis, rhinitis, pharyngitis, otitis media, and even meningitis or encephalitis. Therefore, its mortality rate is high.

1.3 Diagnosis and Differential Diagnosis

The clinical manifestations of influenza are not typical, so it is very easy to be confused it with common cold or acute respiratory infection. Therefore, influenza needs to be diagnosed by integrating epidemic history and clinical symptoms. Check Table 1.1 for key points of differential diagnosis of influenza and common cold.

1.4 Key Points in Treatment

1.4.1 Common Symptomatic Therapy

The patient should be appropriately quarantined in a well ventilated and sterilized room. And the patient should receive bed rest, drink more water, and be supplemented with appropriate nutrition and vitamins. After intake of food, the oral cavity should be rinsed with warm boiled water or warm water with salt. The patient should raise awareness of keeping oral cavity and nasal cavity clean. If systemic symptoms are obvious, anti-infection therapy should be administered.

1.4.2 Anti-viral Therapy

Anti-viral therapy should be administered early.

1.4.3 Use of Antibiotics

The cold is commonly caused by virus. When the symptoms are serious or complications occur, timely clinic visit is recommended. If bacterial infection or complication is definitively diagnosed, antibiotics can be used with professional guidance.

J. Wang
Affiliated First Hospital, Xinjiang Medical University,
Urumuqi, Xinjiang, China
e-mail: jeanw1265@163.com

H. Li (ed.), *Radiology of Influenza*, DOI 10.1007/978-94-024-0908-6_1

Table 1.1 Key points for differential diagnosis of influenza from cold

Key points	Influenza	Cold
Infectivity	Class C infectious disease	Non-infectious disease
Seasonal prevalence	Obvious seasonal prevalence (from Nov. to Mar. of the following year in northern China)	No obvious seasonal prevalence
Fever	Commonly high fever (39–40 °C), possibly with chill	No/mild/moderate fever, with no chill
Duration of fever	3–5 days	1–2 days
Systemic symptoms	Headache, systemic muscle pain and soreness, fatigue	Less symptoms or asymptomatic
complications	Otitis media, pneumonia, and even meningitis or encephalitis	Rare
Illness course	5–10 days	1–3 days
Mortality	High, mostly due to acute aggravation of primary diseases such as lung disease, cardiovascular or cerebrovascular diseases caused by influenza	Low

Etiology of Influenza

2

Jian Wang

Human influenza virus is an enveloped single stranded RNA virus, belonging to the family of Orthomyxoviridae, and can be typed into type A, B, and C. The virus is spherical or filamentous in shape, with a diameter of 80–120 nm. The 3 types of human influenza virus show similar biochemical and biological properties. The viral envelope is composed of three layers: the inner layer of virus nucleocapsid containing nucleocapsid protein (NP), P protein and RNA; the middle layer of virus cyst envelope, composed of a lipoid layer and a layer of membrane protein (MP); and the outer layer of radiating spikes, composed of two different glycoproteins, hemagglutinin (H or HA) and neuraminidase (N or NA). Concerning the inner layer, NP is a type-specific soluble antigen (S antigen) with stable antigenicity. P protein (P1, P2, P3) may be polymerase necessary in transcription and replication of RNA. As for the middle layer, MP is also type-specific with stable antigenicity. And as for the outer layer, both of H and N have antigenicity and subtype specificity. H plays a role in adhering the virus to the surface of sensitive cells, and it can cause agglutination of erythrocytes. N contributes to detaching the virus from the surface of sensitive cells after its replication and it can hydrolyze terminal N- acetylneuraminic acid and mucin of receptor specific glycoprotein on the cell surface. The virus genome, together with the NP on its surface, constitutes the ribonucleoprotein (RNP) complex.

Based on the antigenicity of NP, human influenza virus is typed into type A, B, and C. According to the different H and P antigens, the same type of human influenza virus is further categorized into several subtypes. The antigenic variation of influenza virus refers to the change of H and N antigenic structures, mainly H antigen. Within any subtype of influenza virus, small variations often occur (quantitative), which is known as antigenic drift. The emergence of new subtype (qualitative) due to large antigenic variation of H and/or N antigen is known as antigenic shift, and the new subtype, known as a variant virus strain, can cause pandemic prevalence of influenza. During the 20th century, 4 pandemics of influenza occurred, all of which were caused by type A influenza virus. An obvious alternation exist between an old and a following new subtype of influenza virus. After a new subtype of influenza virus emerges to prevail in a region, the previous old subtype of influenza virus can no longer be isolated in the region. In addition, each subtype of influenza virus produces some variants. Type A influenza virus can be further divided into 16 H subtypes (H1-16) and 9 N subtypes (N1-9). Human influenza is mainly related to subtypes of H1, H2, H3 as well as N1 and N2. Large and small variations also occur in type B influenza virus, but its subtypes have not been definitively divided. And antigenic variation of type C influenza virus has not been reported yet.

Influenza virus is intolerant to heat and can be inactivated at a temperature of 100 °C for 1 min or at a temperature of 56 °C for 30 min. It is sensitive to ultraviolet rays and commonly used disinfectants, such as 1 % formaldehyde, peracetic acid, and disinfectants containing chlorine. Influenza virus is tolerant to low temperature and dryness, and it can survive in vacuum drying environment or at a temperature of under −20 °C. Chicken embryo culture is commonly applied to isolate the virus.

Type A influenza viruses of animal and human share some common antigenic components, but with no cross infection. Generally it can only infect human after antigenic conversion by infecting an intermediate animal host. However, it has been proved recently that some types of avian influenza virus can directly infect human via antigenic variation.

J. Wang
Affiliated First Hospital, Xinjiang Medical University, Urumuqi, Xinjiang, China
e-mail: jeanw1265@163.com

H. Li (ed.), *Radiology of Influenza*, DOI 10.1007/978-94-024-0908-6_2

3 Epidemiology of Influenza

Jian Wang

3.1 Source of Infection

The patients with influenza or latent infection are the main source of its infection, and the infectivity persists for 1–7 days after onset, which is the strongest during the first 2–3 days after onset. Pigs, cattles, horses and other poultries may also spread influenza.

3.2 Route of Transmission

Influenza spreads via droplets in air containing the virus produced by coughing and sneezing of persons with infection. The virus can survive in the air for about half an hour. Healthy individuals can be infected via contacts of hands to mouth or nose following contacts to utensils carrying the virus.

3.3 Susceptible Population

People are generally susceptible to influenza, and certain immunity can be acquired after infection. No cross immunity exists among the three types of influenza virus and among different subtypes of type A influenza virus. And influenza virus may invade an individual repeatedly.

3.4 Prevalence

Influenza occurs suddenly with rapid spread, and its prevalence peaks within 2–3 weeks. Its incidence is high, but only prevails in a short period of time, commonly 6–8 weeks. It commonly spreads along transportation routes, from city to countryside and from working unit to residential area. Influenza occurs all year round, and more commonly in winters and springs. In southern China, its prevalence occurs also in summers and autumns. A small scale prevalence of influenza caused by type A influenza virus occurs every 2–3 years, and a large scale prevalence every 10–15 years. Concerning influenza caused by type B influenza virus, outbreaks or small scale prevalence occur. As for influenza caused by type C influenza virus, its occurrence is sporadic.

J. Wang
Affiliated First Hospital, Xinjiang Medical University,
Urumuqi, Xinjiang, China
e-mail: jeanw1265@163.com

H. Li (ed.), *Radiology of Influenza*, DOI 10.1007/978-94-024-0908-6_3

4 Pathogenesis of Influenza

Jian Wang

Influenza virus can infect various types of cells in human respiratory tract and replicate inside. Viral replication damages its infected cells to cause their apoptosis, which is the underlying mechanism of its pathogenesis. Once influenza virus gains its access to human respiratory tract, it adheres to and penetrates into the epithelial cells for its replication there for 4–6 h. The newly emerging virus particles bud from cell membrane and are released with assistance by neuraminidase to infect adjacent epithelial cells. In such a way, a large quantity of epithelial cells are infected within a short period of time. The infected epithelial cells are then subjected to apoptosis and shedding to cause local inflammatory response as well as systemic toxic symptoms such as acute onset of high fever, systemic soreness and pain, and decreased WBC count. The infected cells can also produce excessive interferon, which may be related to the systemic symptoms. However, viremia does not occur.

The pathological changes of simplex influenza include impaired upper and middle respiratory tract, obviously involved trachea, degenerated ciliated epithelial cells with apoptosis and shedding, detectable inclusion bodies in the cytoplasm, mucosal congestion and edema as well as infiltrated mononuclear cells. However, the layer of basal cells remains intact. About 4–5 days after onset, the basal cells begin to proliferate to form undifferentiated epithelial cells. Two weeks later, ciliated epithelial cells are formed for recovery. Pneumonia induced by influenza virus is pathologically characterized by intrapulmonary extensive hemorrhage in a color of dark red with accompanying edema, bloody secretions in the trachea and bronchi, mucosal congestion, necrosis and shedding of tracheal and bronchial ciliated epithelial cells, submucosal focal hemorrhage, edema and slight inflammatory cells infiltration as well as alveolar fibrin exudates containing neutrophils and mononuclear cells.

J. Wang
Affiliated First Hospital, Xinjiang Medical University,
Urumuqi, Xinjiang, China
e-mail: jeanw1265@163.com

H. Li (ed.), *Radiology of Influenza*, DOI 10.1007/978-94-024-0908-6_4

Diseases Complicating Influenza

5

Jian Wang

5.1 Pneumonia

Pneumonia is the most common complication of influenza, which is inflammation of terminal airway, alveoli and lung interstitium caused by influenza virus infection or secondary bacterial infection. The patients mainly experience clinical symptoms of fever, cough, expectoration, sputum with blood and accompanying chest pain or dyspnea.

5.2 Bronchitis

Bronchitis is an inflammation of bronchial mucosa caused by influenza virus infection or bacterial infection. It is a common disease in infants and young children, with a high incidence in the age group. It commonly occurs secondary to upper respiratory tract infection and is also an early sign of pneumonia. The patients mainly experience cough with/without accompanying increase of tracheal secretion.

5.3 Rhinitis

Rhinitis is an inflammation of mucosa in human nasal cavity, which may be caused by various etiological factors, such as virus, bacteria, allergen, diversifying physical and chemical factors as well as certain systemic diseases. The main pathological changes of rhinitis include congestion, edema, exudation, proliferation, atrophy or necrosis of mucosa in human nasal cavity.

5.4 Pharyngitis

Pharyngitis can be categorized into acute pharyngitis and chronic pharyngitis. Acute pharyngitis is an acute inflammation of pharyngeal mucosa and submucosal tissue, which commonly involves pharyngeal lymphatic tissues. Early inflammation may be confined, but may progress to involve the whole pharyngeal cavity. Its occurrence is more common in alternative periods between autumns and winters as well as between winters and springs.

5.5 Otitis Media

Otitis media is an inflammation involving parts of or whole middle ear (composed of auditory tube, tympanic cavity, tympanic antrum, and mastoid cells), which commonly occurs in children. It can be divided into 2 types, non-purulent and purulent type. Non-purulent type includes secretory otitis media, barotraumatic otitis media, and other otitis media, while purulent type can be further categorized into acute and chronic.

5.6 Encephalitis

Encephalitis is an inflammation caused by invasion of pathogen into brain parenchyma, and the pathogen is the most commonly virus. Other pathogens, such as bacteria, molds, spirochetes, Richettsia, and parasites can also cause encephalitis. In some cases, encephalitis may be allergic disease, such as acute disseminated encephalomyelitis. The clinical term, encephalitis, often refers to viral encephalitis and encephalomyelitis after acute disseminated encephalomyelitis infection.

J. Wang
Affiliated First Hospital, Xinjiang Medical University, Urumuqi, Xinjiang, China
e-mail: jeanw1265@163.com

H. Li (ed.), *Radiology of Influenza*, DOI 10.1007/978-94-024-0908-6_5

5.7 Encephalopathy-Hepatic Steatosis Syndrome

Encephalopathy-hepatic steatosis syndrome, also known as Reye syndrome, is a hepatic or neural complication in patients with type A or B influenza virus infection whose pathogenesis remains unknown and is possibly related to the use of aspirin.

References

Bai RJ, Zhang XL. Medical imaging diagnostics. 3rd ed. Beijing: People's Medical Publishing House; 2010.

Lei BJ. Influenza. In: Peng WW, editor. Studies of infectious diseases. 6th ed. Beijing: People's Medical Publishing House; 2003.

Zhao YR. Influenza. In: Li LJ, editor. Studies of infectious diseases. 2nd ed. Beijing: Higher Education Press; 2011.

6 Radiological Examinations

Xiaochun Zhang

6.1 X-ray

6.1.1 Basic Principles of X-ray

Images of human body can be produced by X-ray onto a screen or a film due to the properties of X-ray, such as its penetration, fluorescent effect and photographic effect, as well as the variances of human tissue in terms of density and thickness. Due to the existence of such variances, X-rays can be absorbed by human tissue in different degrees when it penetrate different human body tissues. Therefore, the dosage of X-ray onto the screen or film is discrepant to show contrasted image on the screen or film.

6.1.2 Application of X-ray in Diagnosis and Assessment of Influenza

X-ray is mainly applied to examine abnormalities of the respiratory system, including trachea, bronchus, lung, pleura, mediastinum and diaphragm. During observing and analyzing lesions in the respiratory system by X-ray, the followings should be paid focused attention: (1) The location and quantity of lesion. (2) The shape and size of lesion. The large flakes of lesion is commonly induced by infections or obstructive atelectasis. The patches of lesion is commonly induced by infectious diseases. And the cords like or network like lesion is commonly induced by interstitial changes. (3) The density and margin of lesion. The density of proliferative lesion is higher than that of exudative lesion. And (4) The effects of lesion on adjacent structures.

Therefore, full knowledge and understanding about basic demonstrations of lesions by X-ray are extremely important for clinical radiologist. They constitute the basis for radiological diagnosis and differential diagnosis of diseases occurring in the respiratory system.

6.1.3 Strengths and Weaknesses of X-ray

X-ray examination has the advantages of simple operation, low cost, favorable mobility for bedside examination of critically ill patients, and low dose of radiation for the examination. It is applicable for observation of lesions in follow-up examinations. However, due to the overlapping tissues or structures, some small lesions at certain body parts may be missed by X-ray examination. In addition, the density resolution by X-ray is comparatively low.

6.2 CT Scan

6.2.1 Basic Principles of CT Scan

CT, i.e., computer tomography, refers to the X-ray emitted by X-ray tube passes through human body after adjusted, focused, and narrowed to fan-shaped beam by a collimator and then received by a detector after adjusted and centralized by another collimator. The X-ray signal received by the detector is attenuated by different tissues in human body. After light/electricity conversion and amplification in a photomultiplier tube and A/D conversion, digital signals are harvested for computer processing to reconstruct transverse sections images. Currently, the commonly used CT scanner have been developed from the previous single layer scanning to spiral, for single row to multi rows, from single source to dual sources, and from single to dual energy.

Currently, CT scan has been widely used in clinical diagnosis, and has great advantages in precise positioning of the lesions and qualitative diagnosis, compared to X-ray. Chest examination is one of the advantages spiral CT scan, allowing the whole lungs to be scanned by 1 mm slice thickness within one breath holding period. In addition, MSCT enables

X. Zhang
Affiliated First Hospital (Xinan Hospital), Third Military Medical University, Chongqing, China
e-mail: zxcylxyr@163.com

H. Li (ed.), *Radiology of Influenza*, DOI 10.1007/978-94-024-0908-6_6

favorable demonstration of the bronchial branches in lungs. Along with continuous development of CT scanner, it has been developed from simplex tomography into high quality multi planar reconstruction (MPR) and a variety of reconstructions, such as surface obscure display (SSD), maximum/minimum density projection (MP), volume rendering (VR) and CT virtual endoscopy (CTE) and CT angiography (CTA). For instances, CT virtual endoscopy can be applied to favorably show the bronchial sub-segment, while the diagnosis by virtual bronchoscopy can be almost as accurate as that by fiberoendoscopy. The reconstruction algorithms have also been developed from 2-dimensional back projection reconstruction into 3-dimensional cone beam back projection reconstruction. In addition to the continual advances of post processing technology, CT scan technology has been developing towards higher quality image, thin thickness, low dose, low noise, and high velocity.

6.2.2 Application of CT Scan in the Diagnosis and Assessment of Influenza

Concerning the diagnosis and therapeutic assessment of influenza and its complications, CT scan is especially appropriate for those patients with persistent lesions or atypical symptoms. By chest CT scan, the lesions may be demonstrated as:

1. Exudative lesion

   By CT scan, the exudation is demonstrated as consolidation and ground glass opacity, which may be small or large flakes of opacity with pulmonary segmental, lobar or diffuse distribution and with air bronchogram in consolidation opacity. It is pathologically based on replacement of most or all air in the alveolar cavity by pathological fluid and cell components, with poorly defined margin. Ground glass opacity is pathologically based on replacement of some air in the alveolar cavity by pathological tissue, with much air remained in the alveolar cavity. Such opacity is commonly observed during the early or absorption stage of alveolar substantial lesions.
2. Proliferative lesion

   Proliferative lesion is radiologically demonstrated as well defined nodules, lumps or large flakes. It may be granuloma, inflammatory pseudoneoplasm and chronic inflammation.
3. Fibrosis

   From the perspective of its development, fibrosis commonly occurs during repair of lung parenchymal damages, which is commonly demonstrated as cords like opacity. Large lesion of fibrosis is demonstrated as patch or lumps like opacity with segmental and lobar distribution as well as irregular shape. In its surrounding lung tissue, constrained pulmonary emphysema is observable. In severe cases, ipsilateral thoracic collapse occurs with ipsilateral shift of the mediastinum. Interstitial lesions are demonstrated as diffuse fibrosis.
4. Pleural effusion

   Pleural effusion is mainly induced by complicating pulmonary edema or pneumonia with pleura involved. By CT scan, the lesions are demonstrated as arch shaped narrow strips in the medial margin of posterior thoracic wall, with uniform liquid density and intact smooth boundary.
5. Pneumothorax and mediastinal emphysema

   Infection of influenza by patients with underlying respiratory diseases may induce wheezing and subsequent increased pressure within lungs, which further causes pneumothorax or mediastinal emphysema. By CT scan, the lesion is demonstrated as highly transparent strip with no lung markings in the lateral lung, with fine linear soft tissue density opacity of the arch shaped visceral pleura inside, which is parallel to the pleura.
6. Mediastinal and axillary lymphadenectasis

   Mediastinal and axillary lymphadenectsis is response to inflammation, commonly with no necrosis or fusion of lymph nodes. CT scan showed slightly high density in the space, with well defined boundary.
7. Plastic bronchitis

   Plastic bronchitis rarely occurs, and its definitive diagnosis is based on bronchoscopy after its aspiration of tree branches like bronchial casts. Pathologically, the lesion is fibrinous exudation with or with no accompanying necrosis. Airway reconstruction following CT scan shows increased density opacity in the lumen.
8. Pulmonary embolism

   Pulmonary embolism rarely occurs.

6.2.3 Strengths and Weaknesses of CT Scan

6.2.3.1 Strengths

CT scan can reveal small lesions. By thin layer scanning, in addition to multi planar reconstruction or 3-dimensional reconstruction, micro-structures of each organ can be clearly shown. Due to its capabilities of thin layer scanning and overlapping reconstruction, the volume effect can be partially limited and the value in detecting and qualifying micro lesions is great.

6.2.3.2 Weaknesses

However, during CT scanning, the radiation dose is comparatively large, and it should not be selected as the examination of choice to diagnose the patients with initial onset of influenza. In addition, it should not be applied for therapeutic assessment in the following-ups of common influenza patients.

6.3 MR Imaging

6.3.1 Basic Principles of MR Imaging

Hydrogen protons, are abundant in human body, with self spinning around its central axis to produce a magnetic field, which has two directions of north and south as well as intensity, known as magnetic moment. Due to the disorderly arrangement of hydrogen protons in human body, their magnetic moments are offset with each other, and human is not magnetic under normal conditions. If hydrogen atom is placed into an externally additional magnetic field (such as access of human body into an MR imaging instrument), the hydrogen protons are rearranged along this externally additional magnetic field, self spinning and rotating along the axis of externally additional magnetic field, which is known as precession. When a hydrogen proton in precession is excited by an energy with the same precession frequency, resonance is produced (commonly RF pulse as the provider of excitation energy). Under the effects of RF pulse, some protons absorb energy to produce phase change and transit into a higher energy state. Therefore, the proton loses its balance in the magnetic field. When the RF pulse ceases, the proton recovers to its original state, which is known as the relaxation. And the period of time for relaxation is known as the relaxation time. During the whole process, the proton in a higher energy state releases energy to produce a signal, which can be detected by a receiving coil around human body. Thus the images are produced after computer processing of the signals.

6.3.2 Application of MR Imaging in the Diagnosis and Assessment of Influenza

MR imaging is mainly applied to detect lesions in the central nervous system that complicate influenza. The commonly detected complications include influenza related encephalopathy, aseptic meningitis, encephalitis and acute necrotizing encephalopathy, and secondary intracranial fungal infection.

6.3.2.1 Influenza Related Encephalopathy

MR imaging displays the deep white matter of the cerebral hemispheres and the basal ganglia (including the thalamus and brainstem tegmentum) with bilaterally symmetric abnormalities.

6.3.2.2 Aseptic Meningitis

Plain MR imaging commonly shows no abnormalities. However, contrast MR imaging occasionally reveals meningeal enhancement, and possible brain and cerebellum enhancements, which are non-specific.

6.3.2.3 Encephalitis and Meningitis

Encephalitis and meningitis are rare complications of influenza. By CT scan, the lesions are demonstrated as low density, while, by MR imaging, low T1 signal but high T2 signal, with slight or no enhancement by contrast imaging.

6.3.2.4 Acute Necrotizing Encephalopathy

MR imaging shows multifocal and symmetric brain lesions. By CT scan, the lesions are demonstrated as low density; while by MR imaging, low T1 signal but high T2 and FLAIR signal. By diffusion weighted imaging (DWI), the bilateral thalamus is shown with central low signal and peripheral high signal; and by ADC, central slightly high signal surrounded by slightly low signal.

6.3.2.5 Secondary Intracranial Fungal Infection

The lesions are radiologically characterized by common fungal infection. Contrast MR imaging demonstrates fungal meningitis as obvious meningeal enhancement; fungal granuloma as round like low T1 signal but high T2 signal, with marginal enhancement by contrast MR imaging.

Due to the favorable imaging effects of MRI on liquid, it is of great help in demonstrating alveolar exudation and pleural effusion in a small quantity as well as in qualitatively identifying the effusion.

6.3.3 Strengths and Weaknesses of MR Imaging

MR imaging has absolute advantages in demonstrating the central nervous system due to its capabilities of multi parameters imaging, 3-dimensional imaging and functional imaging. Therefore, it is the examination of choice for lesions in the central nervous system. For patients incapable of receiving MRI, CT scan acts as the alternative. However, the weakness is its limited application in detecting chest abnormalities.

6.4 Ultrasound

6.4.1 The Principle of Ultrasound

Ultrasound refers to the examination which applies ultrasonic wave with specific direction of bundles transmission, piezoelectric energy conversion device, and variance of sound resistance by different human tissues in imaging of human body. According to the different imaging approaches, it can be divided into A mode, M mode, 2-dimensional, histological, elastic, and 3-dimensional. For patients with influenza, it is mainly applied in quantifying pleural effusion and its following up examinations. Compared to X-ray and CT scan, ultrasound has the advantages of no radiation, repeatability, high sensitivity, convenience for bedside operation, and arbitrary imaging.

6.4.2 Application of Ultrasound in Diagnosis and Assessment of Influenza

For patients with influenza, ultrasound is mainly applied in the diagnosis of pleural effusion. Due to its high sensitivity and specificity as well as positioning accuracy, it can be applied to objectively assess the depth and quantity of pleural effusion as well as to assist puncture positioning. By Color Doppler flow imaging (CDFI), the important blood vessels and alveolar tissues can be protected, with superiorities especially in puncture and drainage of multilocular encapsulated effusion. Meanwhile, it has advantage of simple operations in differentiating pleural effusion, pleural thickening and liquid pneumothorax. It is known that ultrasound findings are the gold standard for the diagnosis of pleural effusion.

6.5 PET/CT

6.5.1 The Basic Principles of PET/CT

By PET, tracer is used to selectively show the changes of tissues and organs in terms of metabolism, physiology, pathology, and biochemistry. However, poorly defined anatomical structures by PET is one of its major weaknesses. However, CT scan, in combination to X-ray, enables attenuated correction of PET images, which greatly reduces the data acquisition time, enhances the image resolution, as well as anatomically localizes and differentiates the lesions on PET images by using CT scan images. PET/CT fundamentally improves the weakness of poorly defined anatomic structures on the images produced by nuclear medicine. Meanwhile, the attenuation co-efficient acquired by CT scan is adopted for all energy attenuation correction of the images by nuclear medicine. Therefore, the images by nuclear medicine can be quantitatively analyzed, which improves the diagnostic accuracy and inter-complementation of functional images and anatomical images.

6.5.2 Application of PET/CT in Diagnosis and Assessment of Influenza

PET/CT is rarely applied in diagnosis and assessment of influenza. However, it is applicable for the patients with incurable chronic lesions or the patients with clinically suspected diagnosis of malignancy or difficulty differentiating inflammation from neoplasm.

6.6 Fibrobronchoscopy

Fibrobronchoscopy is applicable in observing lobar, segmental and sub-segmental bronchial lesions, during which specimen can be collected for biopsy of bacteriological and cytological examinations. It is of help in detecting early lesions in bronchus and defining their quality. Compared to other radiological modalities, fibrobronchoscopy can be applied for both diagnosis and treatment.

Laboratory Test for Diagnosis of Influenza

7

Jie Dai, Hongjun Li, and Li Li

7.1 Laboratory Diagnosis

Laboratory tests for diagnosis of influenza include 4 aspects of examinations, virus culture and isolation, serological test, immunoassay, and molecular biological examination.

7.1.1 Virus Culture and Isolation

Virus culture and isolation is the most common and the most reliable way for the diagnosis of influenza. The specimens for virus culture and isolation include nasopharyngeal swab and oral gargle. Currently, chicken embryo and Madin-Daby canine kidney cells (MDCK cells) are commonly applied for influenza virus culture and isolation.

7.1.1.1 Chicken-Embryo Culture

Chicken-embryo culture is one of the commonly used way for virus culture, which can be applied for virus culture and isolation, titration of virulence, neutralization test as well as preparation of antigen and vaccine. Respiratory viruses, such as orthomyxovirus, paramyxovirus and poxvirus, are sensitive to chicken-embryo culture. Specimens can be harvested from patients for culture and isolation of these viruses. For influenza virus culture and isolation, dual cavities (chicken-embryonic allantonic and amniotic cavities) inoculation is commonly applied.

Generally, chicken embryos aged 9–11 days are applied for amniotic and allantoic cavities inoculation to isolate the virus. Within 24–96 h after inoculation, the fluid in allantoic cavity of chicken embryo should be collected, and the chicken embryo should be rejected within 24 h after death. The chicken erythrocytes are used to test the hemagglutination activity of allantoic fluid or cell culture fluid in order to prove the proliferation and thus the existence of the virus. If the initial virus isolation fails, blind passage for the 2nd generations can be used for another round of test.

7.1.1.2 MDCK Cell Culture

In recent years, with the development of molecular biology technology, the influenza virus isolated via chicken embryo shows different antigenicity from the original specimen, while the antigenicity of influenza virus isolated via MDCK cells resembles to the original specimen. Due to the much higher sensitivity of MDCK cells to the O phase virus strain than chicken embryos, MDCK cells constitute an indispensable host system for isolation of influenza virus, and have gained wide application.

7.1.2 Serological Diagnosis

Serological diagnosis is to detect the level of antibody in serum.

Serological test for influenza virus is based on collection of double sera during the acute stage (within 3 days after onset) and during the convalescent stage (2–4 weeks after onset) for hemagglutination inhibition test, complement binding test, and micro neutralization test for antibody titer. If the antibody titer in the convalescent stage is at least 4 times as high as that in the acute stage, the diagnosis of influenza can be made. Single serum is generally inapplicable for the diagnosis.

Due to the long time for a cycle of serological test and the complex operations, serological diagnosis of influenza is commonly applied in retrospective study, which plays a role in predicting the future prevalence of influenza. However, it contributes little to the early diagnosis of influenza.

J. Dai
Department of Pathology, Capital Medical University, Beijing, China

H. Li (✉) • L. Li
Beijing Youan Hospital, Capital Medical University, Beijing, China
e-mail: lihongjun00113@126.com

H. Li (ed.), *Radiology of Influenza*, DOI 10.1007/978-94-024-0908-6_7

7.1.3 Immunological Diagnosis

7.1.3.1 Immunofluorescent Assay

Immunofluorescent assay is based on the basic principle that the fluorescein labeled antibody binds to the corresponding antigen to form immune complex, which, under a fluorescence microscope, facilitates the observation of virus antigen in cells and its location.

The immunofluorescent assays mainly include direct fluorescent antibody (DFA) test and indirect fluorescent antibody (IFA) test.

Direct Immunofluorescent Assay (DFA)

DFA test adopts monoclonal antibody to target on the antigen of influenza virus. Under a microscope, the respiratory epithelial cells are observed. The finding of virus antigen demonstrates an infection. The test shows a favorable specificity but a low sensitivity.

Indirect Immunofluorescent Assay (IFA)

Due to the binding of antibody to the corresponding antigen to form immune complex, the fluorescein labeled globulin antibody is used to detect the immune complex and therefore speculate the existence of antibody or antigen. By IFA, the known antigen can be used to detect unknown antibody and the known antibody can be used to detect unknown antigen. The test shows both high sensitivity and high specificity, and thus has gained wide application in clinical practice.

7.1.3.2 Immune Colloidal Gold Assay

Immune colloidal gold assay adopts colloidal gold as marker to localize, qualify, and quantify antigen or antibody based on specific binding of antibody to antigen.

Immune colloidal gold assay mainly includes colloidal gold enhanced immunochromatography assay and rapid dot immuno-gold filtration assay. The assay has simple operation with fast result within 10–30 min. In clinic and ICU, it greatly helps in early diagnosis and appropriate treatment.

7.1.4 Molecular Biological Diagnosis

Along with the development of molecular biology, especially the application of polymerase chain reaction technology, molecular biological diagnosis plays an increasingly important role in identifying and typing of influenza virus.

7.1.4.1 Polymerase Chain Reaction (PCR)

Reverse Transcription Polymerase Chain Reaction (RT-PCR)

RT-PCR is a technology integrating reverse transcriptase of RNA and PCR of cDNA. For RT-PCR, the total RNA in tissues or cells can be extracted and the mRNA in it, as template, is reverse transcribed into cDNA by using Oligo (dT) or random primer and reverse transcriptase. The cDNA is then used as template for PCR amplification to obtain the expression of target gene or detected gene. RT-PCR is highly sensitive and specific, which shortens the period time consumed in detection. It is a practical way for early rapid diagnosis of influenza. For detection of RNA virus, RT-PCR is the most commonly used molecular amplification, being capable of identifying the influenza virus and further analyzing its subtype via RNA fragment amplification of the virus genome in the specimen.

Multiple RT-PCR

Multiple RT-PCR is the addition of two or more virus subtypes or specific primers of several viruses in the same PCR system. Based on the length discrepancy of the target fragments, multiple virus subtypes or multiple viruses can be simultaneously detected. It is a rapid and sensitive way of detection with low cost.

Real-Time Fluorescent Quantitative RT-PCR

Real-time fluorescent quantitative RT-PCR is defined as the addition of fluorophores in the RT-PCR system. Based on accumulated fluorescent signals, the whole process of PCR is real-time monitored and the standard curve is used to quantitatively analyze the unknown template. Compared to conventional RT-PCR, real-time fluorescent quantitative RT-PCR has the advantages of high sensitivity, high specificity and rapidity, that enables quantitative analysis of the sample. It has been applied in laboratories specialized in large-scale network surveillance of influenza. Multiple real-time PCR is capable of further analyzing the subtype of influenza virus.

7.1.4.2 Nucleic Acid Sequence Dependent Amplification

Nucleic acid sequence dependent amplification is a rapid isothermal amplification technology with RNA as template that is independent of reverse transcription. It can be performed in collaborations of reverse transcriptase of birds myeloblastoma virus, RNA polymerase of bacteriophage T7, RNase H, two specially designed specific oligonucleotide primers and molecular beacon probe.

Its sensitivity is equivalent to currently used virus cultures, and can be applied to accurately detect the virus, especially detection of the virus RNA.

7.1.4.3 Gene Chip Technology

Gene chip technology is based on the principle that a large number of known nucleotide sequences, as probes, are integrated onto one chip, followed by hybridization with labeled target nucleotide sequences, and the large quantity of gene information in cells or tissues can be detected and analyzed by detecting the hybridization signal.

Gene chip technology has the advantages of high specificity that consumes short period of time. However, due to its weakness of high cost and requirement of complicated device, its application in the detection of influenza virus is still far limited than other examinations.

7.2 Pathological Diagnosis

7.2.1 Influenza A (H1N1)

7.2.1.1 Pathological Changes in the Respiratory System

Generally, it presents as inflammatory responses of the airway, and even lung infection in some severe cases. The main change is primary viral pneumonia, possibly with secondary acute bronchitis, bacterial pneumonia or mixed pneumonia. Autopsies by the CDC of the United States discovered that about 30 % of deaths from influenza A (H1N1) shows concurrent bacterial infection, among which, 50 % is induced by pneumococcus. The change in the late stage of the disease is mainly necrotizing bronchitis, diffuse alveolar damage, pulmonary hemorrhage, intrapulmonary formation of hyaline membrane as well as fibrosis and consolidation of different degrees. In the patients with complications, purulent inflammatory changes are detectable.

The main histopathological changes include congestion and edema of the upper respiratory mucosa, degeneration, necrosis and shedding of bronchial epithelium and gland. The lung lesions are mainly serous and hemorrhagic bronchial pneumonia, with interalveolar septal thickening, interstitial congestion, as well as accompanying infiltration of lymphocytes in a large quantity, serous exudation and focal hemorrhage. In some cases, the condition is accompanied by diffuse alveolar damage, obvious pulmonary edema, apoptosis, necrosis, shedding of the alveolar epithelium, complete alveolar collapse, proliferation of the macrophages and type II alveolar epithelial cells. In the later stage, the pathological changes mainly include necrotizing bronchitis, intrapulmonary formation of hyaline membrane, flakes of hemorrhage of the lung tissue, fibrosis and consolidation of lung tissues in different degrees. In the cases with concurrent bacterial infection, suppurative bronchiolitis, pleuritis, pleural effusion or empyema are shown. Some studies indicated that influenza A (H1N1) may cause high blood coagulation and in some cases, it may cause intrapulmonary minor vascular thrombosis and pulmonary saddle embolism or lobar artery embolism.

7.2.1.2 Pathological Changes of Extrapulmonary Organs

In literature reports, the pathological changes of the extrapulmonary organs in the cases of influenza A (H1N1) are inconsistent. In case reports of some rare severe cases, lymphocytes depletion in bone marrow, spleen and lymph nodes, erythrophagocytosis; acute renal tubular necrosis, myoglobin casts; necrosis, fatty degeneration and cholestasis of the liver; sterile meningitis, myelitis, brain hemorrhage, encephalitis, brain edema, brain herniation; coagulating necrosis of pancreas and spleen; rhabdomyolysis; myocardial infarction, myocarditis, pericarditis and other myocardial damages have been reported. In most literature reports, no obvious abnormalities of extrapulmonary organs have been discovered other than pathological changes of the lungs.

Compared to SARS, another emerging infectious disease, deaths from severe influenza A (H1N1) showed more serious lung hemorrhage, and more obvious damages to the tracheal and bronchial epithelia and glands. In addition to findings by immunohistochemistry and flow cytometry, the virus antigen expression is detected on the pseudostratified ciliated columnar epithelium, tracheal glandular epithelium, bronchiolar epithelial surface, type I and type II alveoli, cytoplasms of vascular endothelial cells and alveolar macrophages. And apoptosis of alveolar epithelial cells is also detected, which may be related to the above mentioned damages.

7.2.2 Human Infected H5N1 Avian Influenza

Currently, autopsies of deaths from human infected H5N1 avian influenza have been rarely reported both nationally in China and internationally. The main findings include pulmonary hemorrhage and consolidation.

7.2.2.1 Pathological Changes of the Respiratory System

The virus infects the nasopharyngeal epithelium and glands, the tonsils, trachea and lung tissue to cause tissue inflammatory responses, such as congestion, edema, and infiltration of perivasrcular lymphocytes. Due to the highest efficiency of virus replication in lungs, the lesions are the most serious there, which are pathologically characterized by pulmonary hemorrhage and necrotizing lesions. The early manifestations include interstitial pneumonia and necrotizing bronchitis; during the progressive stage, with occurrences of diffuse alveolar damage, acute diffuse exudation, accompanying pulmonary edema, multifocal pulmonary hemorrhage, and pulmonary formation of hyaline membrane. During the late stage, the lung tissues are subject to different degrees of fibrosis, organization and consolidation. In the patients with complications, purulent inflammatory changes are detected, including bronchial pneumonia and empyema.

The main histopathological changes include vascular dilation and congestion of alveolar wall in both lungs, filling of pale red edema fluid in the alveolar cavity and different amounts of inflammatory cells, predominantly lymphocytes and macrophages. In addition, syncytoid cells and foam cells are accompanied by formation of hyaline membrane and multifocal hemorrhage. In some areas, the interalveolar septa are subject to thickening with interstitial fibrosis. Some bronchioles and their surrounding alveoli are subject to epithelial detachment, hyperplasia and squamous metaplasia, with alveolar collapse and emphysema of the surrounding lung tissues. In the cases with secondary bacterial infection, the bronchioles and their surrounding alveoli are subject to damages in some areas, with infiltration of neutrophils and formation of small abscesses. In the late stage, the lung tissue shows extensive consolidation.

7.2.2.2 Pathological Changes of Extrapulmonary Organs

H5N1 avian influenza virus shows stronger orientation to tissues than influenza A H1N1 virus. Autopsies and laboratory tests have demonstrated that H5N1 can replicate and reproduce in lymph nodes and other tissues or heart, liver, brain and other organs to involve multiple organs. In addition to primary lung infection, the virus can also directly or indirectly invade the heart, blood vessels, skeletal muscles, liver, kidney and other organs in severe cases. And the patients may experience the symptoms of myocardial fibrous degeneration and necrosis, myocardial interstitial mononuclear cell infiltration, interstitial myocarditis; liver congestion, hepatocytic loose cytoplasm, vesicular fatty degeneration; kidney congestion, renal tubular epithelial cells degeneration and necrosis, cellular casts formation; brain hemorrhage and edema; ascites and pleural effusion; rhabdomyolysis; decreased or absent lymphatic hematopoietic tissue in spleen, thymus, tonsils, and lymph nodes, proliferation and erythrophagocytosis of CD68 positive cells. The virus infection can also cause pulmonary hemorrhage, gingival bleeding, gastrointestinal bleeding and bleeding of other sites.

7.2.3 Human Infected H7N9 Avian Influenza

So far as we know, apart from the animal models of lung infection, no autopsy has been reported about human infected H7N9 avian influenza. Therefore, the clinical management is mainly based on radiological examinations and laboratory tests.

The animal experiments have demonstrated that the lung lesions in mice are the most serious in the cases of human infected H5N1 avian influenza, followed by influenza A H1N1 and human infected H7N9 avian influenza. After infection of H7N9 avian influenza virus, the mice showed comparatively mild responses, with strong ability of self repair of lung tissues. The main lesions mainly include:

1. Shedding of bronchiolar epithelial cell into the lumen and inflammatory cells infiltration around the bronchiolar wall;
2. Interstitial pneumonia, with lung interstitial thickening, congestion and edema of lung, perivascular infiltration of lymphocytes;
3. Pulmonary vasculitis;
4. Diffuse alveolar damage;
5. Pulmonary hemorrhage;
6. Pulmonary interstitial fibrosis.

References

Bai YQ, Xu G, Gong ZL, et al. Human infected highly pathogenic H5N1 avian influenza: autopsy and pathological analysis. Chin J Pathol. 2006;35(9):545–8.

Ciçsek C, Bilgics A. Current approaches to the clinical virologic diagnosis of viral respiratory tract infections. Mikrobiyol Bul. 2003;37(2–3):195–204.

Duan XJ, Li Y, Gong EC. Respiratory pathology of severe influenza A (H1N1): pathological anlaysis of 8 cases. Chin J Pathol. 2011;40(12):825–9.

Ellis J, Iturriza M, Allen R, et al. Evaluation of four real-time PCR assays for detection of influenza A(H1N1)virus. Eum Surveill. 2009;14(22):19–30.

Gao R, Cao B, Hu Y, et al. Human infection with a novel avian-origin influenza A(H7N9)virus. N Engl J Med. 2013;368(20):1888–97.

Li HJ, Li N. Radiology of Influenza A (H1N1): basic theories and clinical practice. Beijing: Tsinghua University Press; 2011.

Lu M, Xie ZG, Gao ZC. Pathological analysis of human infected highly pathogenic H5N1 avian influenza. Chin J Pathol. 2008;37(3):145–9.

Ruixue W, Taubenberger JK.2010. Methods for molecular surveillance of influenza.Expert Rev Anti-infect Ther, 8(5):517–527

Suwannakarn K, Payungporn ST, Samransamruajkit R, et al. Typing(A/B) and subtyping(H1/H3/H5)of influenza A viruses by multiplex real-time RT-PCR assays. J Virol Methods. 2008;152(9): 25–31.

Xia J, Liu F, Wang HL. Detection and typing of influenza virus. Int J Lab Med. 2006;27(6):534–6.

Part II

Clinical Types of Influenza

8 Influenza

Feng Chen, Meiji Ren, and Hongjun Li

8.1 Introduction

Influenza, abbreviated as flu, is an acute respiratory infectious disease caused by influenza virus, which is mainly spread along with droplets with strong infectivity. The influenza virus may cause epidemics or pandemics of influenza and its incidence ranks the first among legally listed infectious diseases. The prevalence of influenza peaks in autumns and winters, with short illness course and self limitation. However, influenza can be complicated by pneumonia or other serious complications that may cause death in populations of infants, young children, the elderly, those with underlying heart and lung disease and those with compromised immunity.

8.1.1 Etiology

In the year of 1971, WHO officially issued the nomenclature system of influenza virus, and the influenza virus is divided into 3 types based on the antigenic properties of the virus nuclear protein since then, type A, type B and type C. Influenza virus is an RNA virus, which is the most stable in an environment with a pH value of 6.5–7.9 and is intolerant to high temperature. It loses its pathogenicity after heated to a temperature of 56 °C for several minutes, and can be inactivated at a temperature of 100 °C for 1 min. In an environment with a low temperature, the virus is more stable, being capable of surviving for more than 1 months at a temperature of 4 °C, and more than 5 months at a temperature of −70 °C. The influenza virus is sensitive to dryness, ultraviolet radiation, and commonly used disinfectants such as ethanol and iodophor.

8.1.2 Epidemiology

8.1.2.1 Source of Infection

The patients with influenza and persons with asymptomatic infection are the main sources of its infection. The infectivity persists from the terminal incubation period to the terminal acute period after onset, and the infectivity is the strongest in the initial 2–3 days after onset.

8.1.2.2 Route of Transmission

Influenza virus exists in the respiratory secretions of the patients or persons with asymptomatic infection and spreads via airborne transmission. By talking, coughing or sneezing, the virus spreads into air along with droplets or aerosols, and causes infection after their being inhaled into susceptible individuals. The virus can also spread via direct or indirect contacts to the mucosa in the oral cavity, nasal cavity, and eyes.

8.1.2.3 Susceptible Population

Populations are generally susceptible to influenza, which is not related to the gender and occupation. After infection, individuals acquire certain immunity. Among influenza virus A, B and C as well as different subtypes of influenza A virus, no cross immunity exists. And influenza virus can be repeatedly infected. After infection, the acquired immunity only persists for a short period of time. Despite of antibodies in the blood, the person can be infected by the same virus again.

8.1.3 Clinical Manifestation

The incubation period of influenza lasts for about 13 days, and several hours in some cases. Its onset is sudden and acute and the patients mainly experience systemic toxic symptoms but inapparant respiratory symptoms. According to the clini-

F. Chen • M. Ren • H. Li (✉)
Beijing Youan Hospital, Capital Medical University, Beijing, China
e-mail: lihongjun00113@126.com

H. Li (ed.), *Radiology of Influenza*, DOI 10.1007/978-94-024-0908-6_8

cal manifestations, influenza can be divided into the following types.

8.1.3.1 Simplex Type

The simplex type is the most common, and is often characterized by sudden onset of aversion to cold and high fever with a body temperature of up to 39–40 °C. Fever is the most important initial sign, often accompanied by headache, systemic muscle and joint soreness and pain, fatigue, poor appetite, and other toxic symptoms. Some patients may experience such symptoms as photophobia and tears. Other symptoms, such as nasal obstruction, runny nose, sore throat, voice hoarseness and other respiratory symptoms also show at the onset.

8.1.3.2 Pneumonia Type (Primary Influenza Virus Pneumonia)

Pneumonia type may be secondary to the simplex type or occurs as primary influenza virus pneumonia, which is caused by spread of influenza virus from upper respiratory tract to lower respiratory tract. The pneumonia type commonly occurs in the elderly, children, patients with underlying heart and/or lung disease, pregnancies, and individuals with compromised immunity. The main manifestations include persistent high fever, difficulty breathing, cynosis, severe cough, expectoration of foamy mucous sputum or purulent sputum, expectoration of sputum with blood.

8.1.3.3 Toxic Type

The toxic type of influenza is extremely rare in clinical practice, which is caused by invasion of influenza virus into the central nervous system and cardiovascular system, with manifestations of toxic symptoms. Clinically, the patients experience symptoms of encephalitis or meningitis, with high fever, coma, delirium, convulsions, and even meningeal irritation sign and diffuse intravascular coagulation that indicate serious condition.

8.1.3.4 Gastrointestinal Type

The gastrointestinal type of influenza is common in children, and is mainly characterized by nausea, vomiting, diarrhea, and abdominal pain.

8.1.4 Radiological Demonstration

8.1.4.1 Primary Influenza Virus Pneumonia

Chest X-ray demonstrates mainly interstitial pneumonia and bronchial pneumonia, initially with poorly defined thickening of the lung markings, predominantly both lower lung field significantly; increased density of the lung markings resembling to GGO. During the progressive stage, the lung fields are demonstrated with grid like opacity and network like nodular opacity, with the nodules smaller than 5 mm. Such signs may be concurrently shown with thickened and blurry lung markings, with a distribution in both lower lung fields and around the hilum. In the late stage, cystic changes are shown in different sizes due to bronchiolar inflammatory occlusion in honeycomb like lungs, in addition to shrinkage of lungs, elevated diaphragm and shift of interlobar fissure. CT scan demonstrates small nodular opacity, GGO, tree-bud sign and mosaic like perfusion as well as interlobular septal thickening, subpleural line, adjacent pleural thickening, and pleural effusion.

8.1.4.2 Complication of Bacterial Pneumonia

Chest X-ray shows alveolar pneumonia (lobar pneumonia) or bronchial pneumonia (lobular pneumonia). Alveolar pneumonia is mainly demonstrated as lobar consolidation opacity with high homogeneous density or consolidation opacity with high homogeneous density occupying part of lung lobe, possibly with air bronchogram. Due to the different location of the lung lesions, the radiological demonstrations are accordingly different, with one or multiple lung lobes involved. Bronchial pneumonia is demonstrated as thickened lung markings, with poorly defined nodular opacity in diameters of 6–8 mm or poorly defined flakes of opacity. Large poorly defined patch of opacity with uneven density is the result of overlapping lesions of lobular alveolitis. Bronchial obstruction by mucus is demonstrated as lobular atelectasis or focal emphysema in the diseased area. Bronchiolar occlusion may cause a small triangular shaped lesion of atelectasis. The lesions are commonly located in the medial parts of both lower lung fields, with more lesions in the posterior lung lobe than in the anterior lung lobe. And the lesions distribute along bronchi, with smooth air flow in the segmental and lobar bronchi. Terminal bronchiolar mucosa may be subject to congestion, edema and inflammatory exudation to cause obstructive emphysema, which is demonstrated as increased transparency of both lungs, thoracic extension, widened intercostal space, lowered and flat diaphragmatic muscle. CT scan demonstrates consolidation with uniform shape, lobar distribution and inner air bronchogram as well as poorly defined nodular and patches of opacity in different sizes that distributes along bronchial bundles. In addition, lobular pulmonary atelectasis and focal emphysema are also shown by CT scan.

8.2 Typical Cases

Case 1

[Brief Case History]

A 7-years-old boy complained of fever and cough for 2 days, with the highest body temperature of 37.7 °C. Laboratory tests revealed WBC count 4.21×10^9/L, and nucleic acid of influenza virus positive.

[Radiological demonstration] Fig. 8.1

[Diagnosis] Influenza virus pneumonia

[Discussion]

This is a case of influenza virus pneumonia, demonstrated by chest X-ray as interstitial inflammation in both lungs. Chest X-ray demonstrates primary influenza virus pneumonia mainly as interstitial pneumonia and bronchial pneumonia, early with poorly defined but enhanced lung markings, predominantly in bilateral lower lung fields. In addition, the lung markings show an increased density, resembling to GGO. During the progressive stage, the lung fields are demonstrated with reticular opacity and reticular nodular opacity, with nodules smaller than 5 mm. Such opacities may be concurrently demonstrated with poorly defined but enhanced lung markings. The lesions are commonly located in both lower lung fields and around the hilum. Chest CT scan demonstrates small nodular opacity in lungs, GGO, tree-buds sign and mosaic like perfusion, interlobular septal thickening, subpleural line, adjacent pleural thickening and pleural effusion. By radiology, the condition of this case was mild, present difficulty for the diagnosis, which depended on rich experience of the radiological clinician.

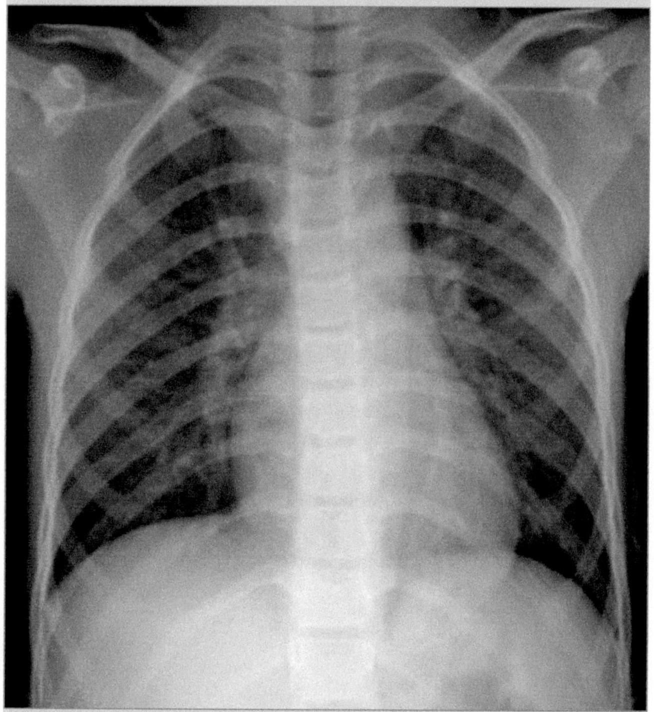

Fig. 8.1 Chest X-ray demonstrated thickened lung markings as well as spots and small flakes of opacities along lung markings in the middle and medial parts of both lung fields

In this case, influenza virus pneumonia manifested as interstitial pneumonia should be differentiated from other viral pneumonia, such as hand-foot-mouth virus pneumonia and measles virus pneumonia. The initial lesions of hand-foot-mouth virus pneumonia are mainly interstitial changes with an extensive distribution and possible involvement of each lung lobe. The lesions commonly distribute bilaterally, with enhanced and deranged lung markings in both lungs as well as common grid like and cords like opacity. Along with the progression of the lesions, chest X-ray demonstrates changes of the lesions, with peripheral spread of the lobular lesions along bronchi and inflammatory consolidation of alveoli and adjacent lung tissue. The lesion may also invade alveolar duct, alveolar sac and alveoli in the lung lobule to cause lobular inflammatory exudation, demonstrated as small patches of increased density opacity confined within lung lobe or segment. There are more exudation opacities in the upper lung lobes than in the lower lung lobes and more in the right lung lobes than in the left lung lobes. Chest X-ray demonstrates measles virus pneumonia as flakes or diffuse ground glass opacity and/or thickened bronchovascular bundles. CT scan demonstrates poorly defined centrilobular nodules, ground glass opacities, interlobular septal thickening as well as lobular or segmental consolidations. Adenovirus pneumonia is demonstrated as thickened and blurry lung markings as well as small nodular opacities along lung markings in the middle and medial parts of bilateral middle and lower lung fields, possibly with fused lesions.

The radiological demonstrations of influenza virus pneumonia resemble to those of other viral pneumonia, and the radiological diagnosis of the primary disease is, therefore, challenging. The diagnosis can be defined based on laboratory tests.

Case 2

[Brief Case History]

A 6-years-old boy complained of fever and cough with skin rashes for 6 days, with the highest body temperature of 38.9 °C. Laboratory tests revealed WBC count $2.26 \times 10^9/L$, PCO_2 42.6 mmHg, and PO_2 86.5 mmHg; the nucleic acid of influenza virus positive.

[Radiological demonstration] Fig. 8.2

[Diagnosis] Influenza virus pneumonia.

[Discussion]

This case of influenza virus pneumonia is typically as virus pneumonia. Chest X-ray demonstrates primary influenza virus pneumonia as interstitial pneumonia and bronchial pneumonia, with initial radiological signs of enhanced but poorly defined lung markings, predominantly in bilateral lower lungs. The lung markings also show increased density resembling to ground glass opacity. During the progressive stage, the lung fields are demonstrated with reticular and reticular nodular opacities, with nodules smaller than 5 mm. Such opacities can be concurrently demonstrated with enhanced but poorly defined lung markings. The lesions commonly distribute in both lower lung fields and around the hilum. The demonstrations by CT scan are diversifying and overlapping, including small nodules in lungs, tree-buds sign with sporadic and centrilobular distribution, ground glass opacity with lobar distribution, diffuse ground glass opacities accompanied by thick interstitial change as well as interlobular septal thickening, subpleural line, adjacent pleural thickening, and pleural effusion. The radiological findings are in consistency with the histopathological demonstrations.

The disease should be mainly differentiated from measles virus pneumonia, pulmonary alveolar pneumonia and allergic pneumonia. Chest X-ray demonstrates measles virus pneumonia as flakes or diffusely distributed GGO and/or thickened bronchovascular bundles. By CT scan, measles virus pneumonia is demonstrated as poorly defined centrilobular nodules, ground glass opacity, interlobular septal thickening as well as lobular or segmental consolidation opacities. Bacterial pneumonia is mainly demonstrated as alveolar pneumonia or bronchial pneumonia. Alveolar pneumonia is mainly demonstrated as lobar consolidation opacity with high uniform density or consolidation opacity occupying part of lung lobe, with air bronchogram inside. Bronchial pneumonia is demonstrated as thickened lung markings, with poorly defined nodular opacity or poorly defined flakes of opacity. Allergic pneumonitis is a non-asthmatic allergic lung disease caused by a group of different allergens. Chest X-ray may show no abnormalities or diffuse interstitial fibrosis, commonly with bilateral patches or nodular infiltration, thickening of the bronchial lung markings or small acinar like changes. CT scan shows thickened bronchovascular thickening, poorly defined small patches of and ground glass opacities along the bronchovascular bundles. The demonstrations by CT scan are irregular, possibly with inconsistencies between radiological findings and clinical symptoms.

Unlike bacterial pneumonia, the radiological signs of viral pneumonia may be inconsistent with the clinical symptoms. Therefore, radiological diagnosis of primary virus pneumonia is challenging and the diagnosis can be defined based on the laboratory tests.

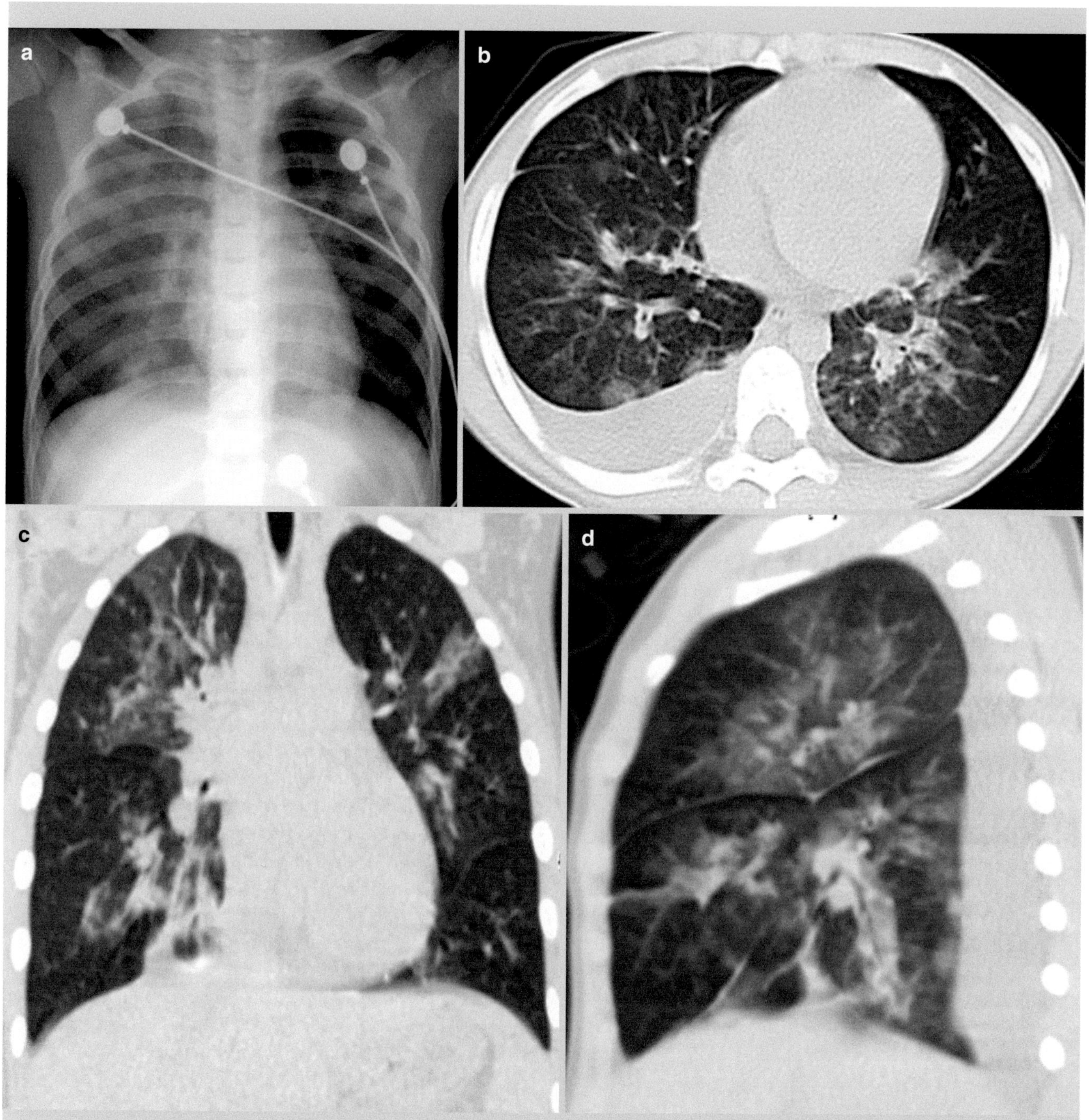

Fig. 8.2 Chest X-ray showed thickened lung markings, decreased transparency of the right lung field, sporadic flakes of poorly defined opacities in both lung fields (**a**). CT scan demonstrated ground glass opacities along bronchovascular bundles in both lungs and right pleural effusion (**b–d**)

Case 3

[Brief Case History]

A 7-years-old boy complained of fever and cough for 2 days, with aversion to cold and the highest temperature of 39.4 °C. Laboratory tests revealed WBC count 15.4×10^9/L; the nucleic acid of influenza virus positive.

[Radiological demonstration] Fig. 8.3

[Diagnosis] Influenza complicated by bacterial pneumonia.

[Discussion]

This is a case of influenza complicated by bacterial pneumonia, with typical signs of lobar pneumonia. Lobar pneumonia is commonly caused by Streptococcus pneumoniae, with sudden and acute onset and a short course of illness. Chest X-ray demonstrates bacterial pneumonia as alveolar pneumonia (lobar pneumonia) or bronchial pneumonia (lobular pneumonia). Alveolar pneumonia is mainly demonstrated as lobar consolidation with high uniform density or consolidation with high uniform density occupying a part lung lobe, with air bronchogram inside. The lesions at different sites show different radiological signs, with lesions involving one lung lobe or multiple lung lobes. Bronchial pneumonia is demonstrated as thickened lung markings, with poorly defined nodular or flakes of opacity in a diameter of 6–8 mm. And the large poorly defined patches of opacity with uneven density is actually overlapping opacities of multiple lobular alveolitis. Occlusion of bronchi by mucus is demonstrated as lobular atelectasis or focal emphysema, while occlusion of bronchiole causes radiological sign of a small triangle shaped lung atelectasis. The lesions are commonly located in the medial parts of both lower lung fields, with more lesions in the posterior lung lobe than in the anterior lung lobe, which distribute along bronchial branches with smooth air flow in the segmental and lobar bronchi. Congestion, edema and inflammatory exudation of terminal bronchiolar mucosa may cause obstructive emphysema, which is demonstrated as increased transparency of both lung fields, extended thorax, widened intercostal space, and lowered flat diaphragm. CT scan demonstrates uniform shaped consolidations with lobar distribution, with air bronchogram inside, and poorly defined nodular and patches of opacity in different sizes along bronchical bundle as well as lobular atelectasis or focal emphysema.

It should be mainly differentiated from viral pneumonia, Klebsiella pneumonia and mycoplasma pneumonia.

Chest X-ray demonstrates viral pneumonia mainly as interstitial pneumonia and bronchial pneumonia. During its early stage, chest X-ray demonstrates enhanced but poorly defined lung markings, predominantly in the both lower lung fields, with increased density like GGO. During the progressive stage, the lung fields are demonstrated with reticular opacity and reticular nodules, which mainly distribute in both lower lung fields and around the hilum, with a diameter of less than 5 mm. During the advanced stage, bronchiolar inflammatory occlusion causes cystic changes in different sizes, with honeycomb like lung. The lung is demonstrated with shrinkage, elevated diaphragm and shift of interlobar fissure. CT scan demonstrates small nodules, ground glass opacity, tree-buds sign and mosaic like perfusion. Klebsiella pneumonia is an acute lung inflammation caused by Klebsiella pneumoniae, which commonly occurs in populations of those with chronic alcoholism or malnutrition and the elderly. Chest X-ray demonstrations can be classified into 3 types: increased lung markings type; lobular type or diffuse pneumonia type; and lobar consolidation type or lung abscess type. Compared to chest X-ray, CT scan can more favorably display the lesions. In its early stage, Klebsiellar pneumonia is demonstrated with lobular sporadic distribution of patches or irregular dense opacities, which involve multiple lung segments and fuse rapidly to show lobar consolidation in the right upper lung lobe. Due to the thick exudated fluid from the lesion, the interlobar fissure is demonstrated to drop. The lesions are susceptible to necrosis, followed by formation of lung abscess, which is commonly multiple small cavities with a diameter of less than 2 cm. The healing proce ss of these cavities is long, commonly with residual extensive fibrosis. Mycoplasma pneumonia is an acute respiratory infection and pneumonia caused by Mycoplasma pneumonia, with common occurrence in both children and adults. Most of the patients show cold agglutination test positive. In its early stage, chest X-ray demonstrates increased poorly defined lung markings and blurry cloud like or homogenous opacities, commonly in the middle and lower lung fields. Such opacities adjacent to the hilum are dense, and its density gradually lightens along with its distance from the hilum, with poorly defined boundary and involvement of partial lung lobe. Mycoplasma pneumonia with lobar lesion can not be differentiated from lobar pneumonia induced by other pathogenic bacteria. Chest CT scan mainly shows ground glass like opacity in lungs, nodular or small patches of consolidation with air cavity, thickened bronchovascular bundle, buds-in-tree sign, large consolidation as well as accompanying mediastinal lymphadenectasis and pleural effusion.

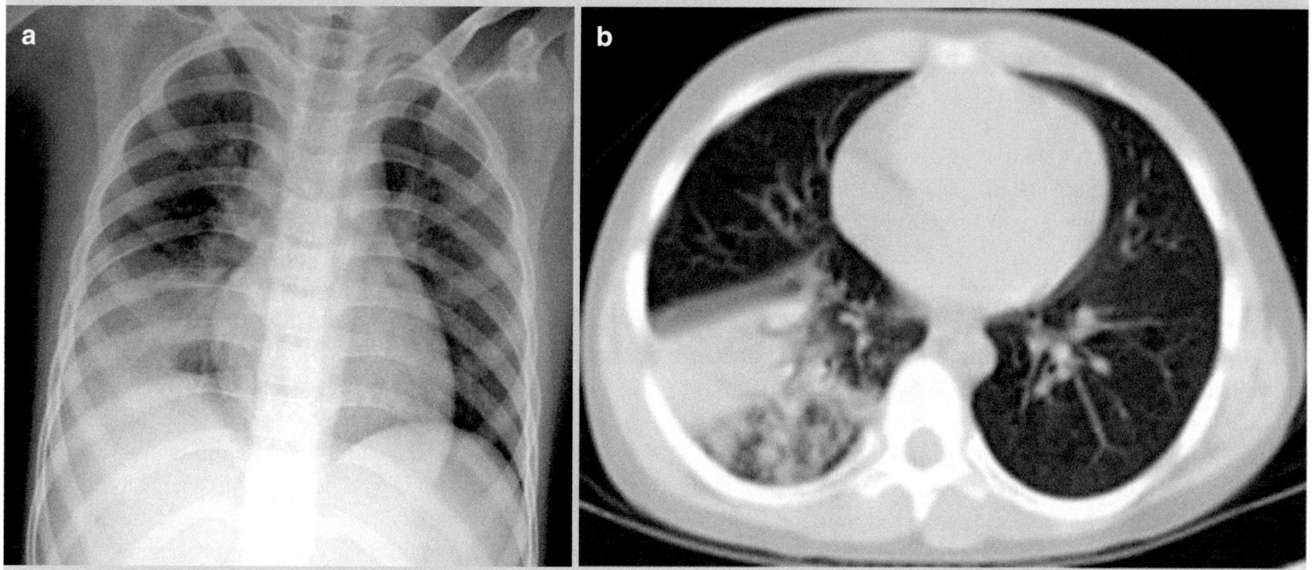

Fig. 8.3 Chest X-ray demonstrated thickened lung markings in both lungs, decreased transparency of the right lower lung field, and poorly defined flakes of opacities in the right lower lung (**a**). CT scan demonstrated wedge shaped consolidation opacity in the right lower lung lobe, with its sharp end pointing to the hilum, air bronchogram inside and surrounding poorly defined small patches of opacities (**b**)

Case 4

[Brief Case History]

A 22-years-old woman, pregnant for 38 weeks, complained of fever and aversion to cold for 2 days with the highest body temperature of 39.1 °C. Laboratory test revealed WBC count 19.48×10^9/L, PCO_2 33.8 mmHg, PO_2 43.6 mmHg, SaO_2 80.9 %; the nucleic acid of influenza virus positive.

[Radiological demonstration] Fig. 8.4

[Diagnosis] Influenza complicated by ARDS.

[Discussion]

Different populations with influenza, show different clinical manifestations, and the special populations include children, the elderly, the pregnancy and those with compromised immunity. In the middle or late stage of pregnancy, women, after infected by influenza virus, experience the symptoms of fever and cough, with vulnerability to pneumonia. The condition rapidly progresses into dyspnea, hypoxemia and even ARDS, with outcomes of miscarriage, premature delivery, fetal distress and intrauterine fetal death. In addition, it may induce aggravation of the underlying diseases, with occurrence of death in severe cases. In this case, the patient was a young woman during her pregnancy, who was diagnosed with influenza complicated by ARDS and death occurred after active treatment due to multiple organs failure.

ARDS is the typical manifestation of advanced stage acute lung damage, which is basically diffuse capillary damage of lung with increased permeability due to intrapulmonary or extrapulmonary serious disease. Its pathological changes include pulmonary edema, hyaline membrane formation and pulmonary atelectasis, with clinical manifestations of acute respiratory failure syndrome characterized by progressive respiratory distress and intractable hypoxemia. The radiological abnormalities of ARDS are related to leakage of edema fluid containing a large amount of protein and its filling into the alveolar cavity after damage to the alveolar epithelium or diffuse damage to alveolar wall. And its staging by radiology is closely related to the pathological changes, including the exudative stage, the proliferative stage and the fibrosis stage, with intercorrelationship and overlapping. Chest X-ray commonly demonstrates diffuse opacity in both lungs, and detectable lesions of the underlying disease, e.g. severe pneumonia induced by a variety of pathogens. CT scan demonstrates uneven distribution of the lesions: (1) with almost no abnormality in the gravity independent region (e.g. supine, anterior thoracic cavity); (2) with GGO in the anterior and middle thoracic cavity; and (3) with consolidation in the gravity dependent region.

In the cases with no capillary damage in lung, the patches of opacities evenly distribute in both lungs, with no gravity dependent lesions and no gravity dependent changes of the lesions. Such a phenomenon facilitates its differential diagnosis from other lung infections. In the advanced stage of ARDS, radiology demonstrates twisted and stretching of the bronchi, shrinkage of lung segment or lobe, grid like opacity, cords like opacity, honeycomb like opacity, and even honeycomb like lung in severe cases.

It should be mainly differentiated from viral pneumonia, bacterial pneumonia and pulmonary edema. Chest X-ray demonstrates viral pneumonia mainly as interstitial pneumonia and bronchial pneumonia. In its early stage, chest X-ray demonstrates enhanced but poorly defined lung markings, predominantly both lower lung fields, with increased density like GGO. In its progressive stage, the lung fields are demonstrated with reticular opacity or reticular nodules and the nodules commonly distribute in the both lower lung fields and around the hilum, with a diameter of less than 5 mm. It its advanced stage, bronchiolar inflammatory occlusion causes cystic changes in different sizes to show honeycomb like lung, with shrinkage of lung, elevated diaphragm and shift of interlobar fissure. CT scan demonstrates small nodular opacity, ground glass opacity, tree-buds sign and mosaic like perfusion in lungs. Chest X-ray demonstrates bacterial pneumonia mainly as alveolar pneumonia or bronchial pneumonia. Alveolar pneumonia is demonstrated as lobar consolidation with high uniform density or consolidation with high uniform density occupying part of lung lobe, with air bronchogram inside and one or multiple lung lobes involved. Bronchial pneumonia is demonstrated as thickened lung markings, poorly defined nodular or flakes of opacity in a diameter of 6–8 mm. Bronchial occlusion by mucus can be demonstrated as lobular atelectasis or focal emphysema in the diseased area. The lesions are commonly located in the medial part of both lower lung fields, with more in the posterior lung lobe than in the anterior lung lobe, that distribute along bronchial branches. And the segmental and lobar bronchi show smooth air flow. CT scan demonstrates consolidations with uniform shape and lobar distribution, with air bronchogram inside, and poorly defined nodular or patches of opacities of different sizes along bronchial bundles as well as lobular atelectasis and focal emphysema. Pulmonary edema and acute or chronic systolic or diastolic heart dysfunction due to various etiological factors can lead to increased pressure in the pulmonary vein and pulmonary capillaries as well as pulmonary congestion. The liquid firstly accumulates in the perivascular sheath in lungs and interlobular space to cause pulmonary interstitial edema, which then flow into the alveolar cavity to cause pulmonary parenchyma edema. Chest X-ray demonstrates interstitial edema as thickened, deranged and re-ranged lung markings, thickened but poorly defined vascular markings in both upper lung fields, enlarged and dense hilar opacities in both lungs, thickened and dilated but poorly defined vascular markings in the middle and medial parts of both lung fields. However, chest X-ray demonstrates interstitial edema with fine vascular markings in peripheral lung field and well defined peripheral lung field. Its further progression can be demonstrated with flakes of opacity in both lungs with butterfly wing like shape and concentric distribution. Chest X-ray demonstrates alveolar edema as initially poorly defined flakes of opacities in different sizes with sporadic distribution in both lungs. Along with its progression, chest X-ray demonstrates large flakes of high density opacity after fusion, which extends from the hilum to the peripheral lung with gradually light density, in typical butterfly wing like sign.

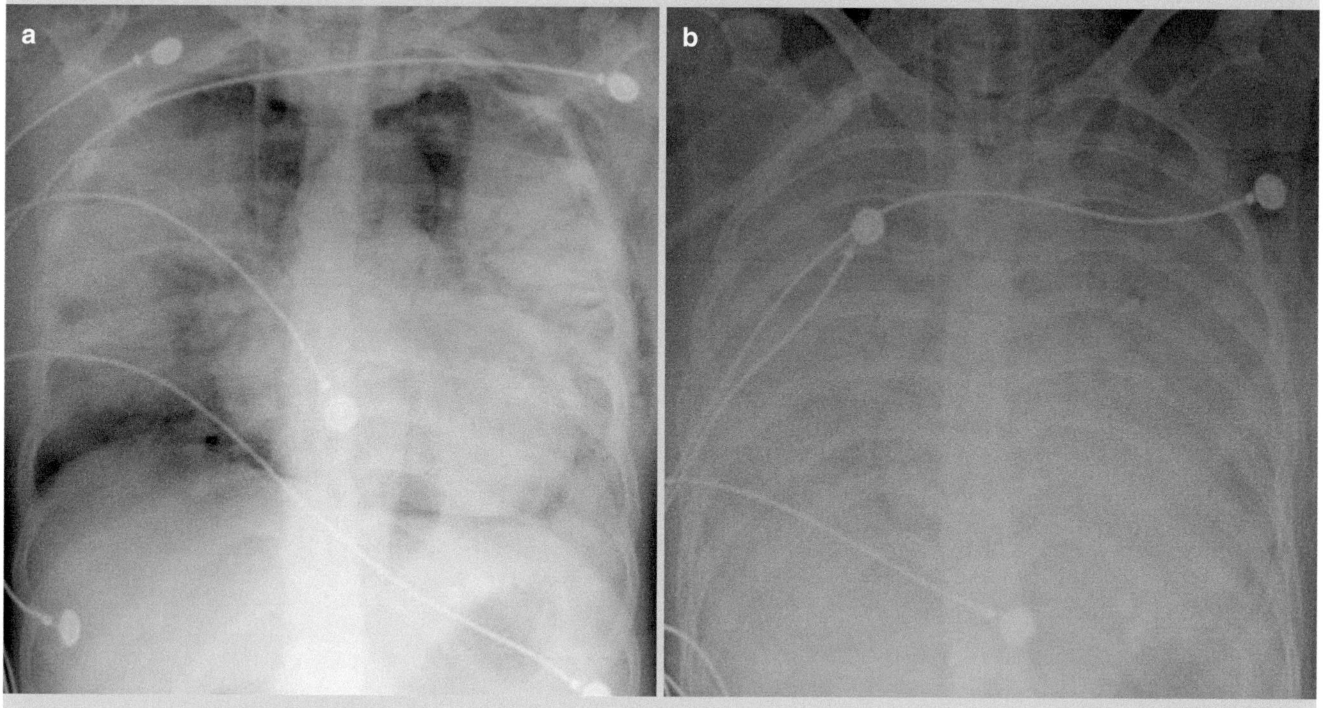

Fig. 8.4 Chest X-ray demonstrated decreased transparency of both lung fields and large consolidation opacity in both lungs, with air bronchogram inside (**a**). Reexamination after treatment for 2 days showed that absence of lung markings in both lungs, further decreased transparency of both lung fields, and diffuse high density in both lungs (**b**)

References

Branch of Respiratory Diseases, Chinese Medical Association. Diagnostic criteria of acute lung injury and acute respiratory distress syndrome. Chin J Tubercu Respir. 2000;23(4):203.

Gattinoni L, Caironi P, Pelosi P, et al. What has computed tomography taught us about the acute respiratory distress syndrome? Am J Respir Crit Care Med. 2001;164(9):1701–11.

Li TY. Imaging diagnosis of interstitial pneumonia. J Pract Med Imaging. 2003;4(1):1–2.

Li XQ, Li HJ. Chest X-ray demonstrations of pediatric hand-foot-mouth disease complicated by pneumonia. Radiol Pract. 2014;29(8):937–41.

Nambu A, Ozawa K, Kobayashi N, et al. Imaging of community-acquired pneumonia: Roles of imaging examinations, imaging diagnosis of specific pathogens and discrimination from noninfectious diseases. World J Radiol. 2014;6(10):779–93.

Reittner P, Ward S, Heyneman L, et al. Pneumonia: high-resolution CT findings in 114 patients. Eur Radiol. 2003;13(3):515–21.

9 Influenza A (H1N1)

Hongjun Li, Li Li, Bailu Liu, Min Li, Ping Li, and Yinglin Guo

9.1 Introduction

9.1.1 The History of Its Prevalence and Impacts

In March 2009, an outbreak of human infected swine influenza, first name by WHO, occurred in Mexico that rapidly spread worldwide. On Apr 30, 2009, the WHO, the United Nations Food and Agriculture Organization and the World Organization for Animal Health agreed to use the name of influenza A (H1N1), which was then used in bulletins issued by Ministry of Health in China.

In the context of international financial crisis, influenza A (H1N1) spread worldwide, posing new variables to the already bleak world economic outlook. So far, strict measures for prevention and control of influenza A (H1N1) have been adopted in China. To some extent, thanks to the transparent information system on infectious diseases as well as emergency precaution and management mechanism established by the Chinese government, the spread of influenza A (H1N1) in China has been well controlled.

H. Li (✉) • L. Li
Beijing Youan Hospital, Capital Medical University, Beijing, China
e-mail: lihongjun00113@126.com

B. Liu • P. Li
Affiliated Second Hospital, Harbin Medical University, Harbin, Heilongjiang, China

M. Li
Suzhou Fifth People's Hospital, Suzhou, Jiangsu, China

Y. Guo
Taiping People's Hospital, Daowai District, Harbin, Heilongjiang, China

9.1.2 Etiology and Epidemiology

The first case of influenza A (H1N1) in the United States was confirmatively diagnosed via laboratory diagnosis on Apr 15, 2009. The researchers discovered that influenza A (H1N1) virus is a complex virus composed of 4 variant viruses, including 1 avian influenza virus, 1 common influenza virus and 2 swine influenza viruses that widely spread in pigs. Meanwhile, the researchers proved that rearrangement and recombination of influenza A (H1N1) virus genes commonly and extensively exist. Currently, the pathogenesis of influenza A (H1N1) virus has attracted focused attention by scholars both internationally and within China. It has been demonstrated that apoptosis of host cells induced by influenza A (H1N1) virus contributes to its pathogenesis. Many studies have proved that influenza A (H1N1) virus induces apoptosis that is mediated via Caspase approach, which can be regulated by multiple channels, multiple factors and multiple genes. It has been also proved that influenza A (H1N1) virus induces apoptosis with a complex process.

On Apr 30, 2009, influenza A (H1N1) was listed as a class B infectious disease and an infectious disease receiving frontier health inspection and quarantine, which should then be managed as the class A infectious diseases in China.

For the epidemic of influenza A (H1N1), the patients with influenza A (H1N1) are the source of its infection and the virus spreads from person to person along with respiratory aerosols and droplets. The populations are generally susceptible to the infection, and the young and middle-aged adults are especially vulnerable. Factors influencing its prevalence include host factors, virus factors, social conditions, health care insurance, and other natural and social factors.

9.1.3 Clinical Manifestations and Diagnosis

Human infected influenza A (H1N1) commonly has an incubation period of 1–7 days, which is comparatively longer than common influenza and human infected avian influenza.

H. Li (ed.), *Radiology of Influenza*, DOI 10.1007/978-94-024-0908-6_9

The symptoms of influenza A (H1N1) range from normal body temperature and mild upper respiratory infection to severe or fatal pneumonia. Most of the patients experience typical influenza like symptoms and self heal. Severe and death cases are mostly caused by occurrence of complications, including preliminary viral pneumonia and secondary bacterial pneumonia.

The most common symptoms include cough, fever, sore throat, runny nose, nasal obstruction, cough, expectoration, headache, systemic soreness, and fatigue. Some patients may experience vomiting and/or diarrhea. Mild upper respiratory symptoms rarely occur, but no fever. And the physical signs include pharyngeal congestion and enlarged tonsils.

Its diagnosis is mainly based on the epidemiology, clinical manifestations and etiological examination. The inpatients show increased or decreased WBC count; severe cases commonly show decreased total WBC count, lymphocytes, and platelets. Other diagnostic examinations include serological test, virus isolation (such as throat swab as well as specimens of oral gargle, nasopharyngeal or tracheal aspirates, sputum, and lung tissue), reverse transcription polymerase chain reaction (RT-PCR) are also important ways for the diagnosis of influenza A (H1N1). Early detection and early diagnosis are the keys for its prevention, control and effective treatment.

9.1.4 Radiological Demonstrations

9.1.4.1 Nervous System

Japanese researchers have discovered that influenza virus infection in some children may further cause encephalitis due to its invasion into their central nervous system.

By craniocerebral CT scan, the patients with influenza A (H1N1) complicated by encephalitis are mostly demonstrated with symmetric low density in bilateral basal ganglia, bilateral thalamus, and bilateral white matter of frontal brain; and some patients may show no obvious abnormalities. Brain MR imaging shows symmetric long T1 and long T2 signals at the above mentioned sites. FLAIR and DWI often demonstrate high signal. In some patients, cerebellum is demonstrated with involvement. By contrast scan or imaging, meningeal enhancement may be demonstrated.

9.1.4.2 Chest

The patients with influenza A (H1N1) rarely show chest abnormalities. And the common abnormalities by chest radiology include GGO and consolidation. The lung lesions in adult lungs commonly distribute in the lower fields of both lungs, but no characteristic distribution in pediatric patients. The focal, multiple or diffuse lung lesions may be within one lung or both lungs, resembling to SARS and other viral pneumonia. The radiological signs of pulmonary nodules, interstitial thickening, patches of opacity around bronchus, air trapping sign, and pleural effusion are rare. Severe and critical cases of influenza A (H1N1) can be complicated by pulmonary embolism. Being different from other lung infections, the cases of influenza A (H1N1) rarely show enlarged lymph nodes, with no central lobular nodule and tree-buds sign by MSCT.

Compared to common chest X-ray, CT scan is more sensitive to GGO and shows higher accuracy in detecting the distribution of lesions. However, common chest X-ray has the advantage of simple operational procedures, especially bedside chest X-ray for critical cases of influenza A (H1N1).

9.1.4.3 Abdomen

The patients with severe influenza A (H1N1) may subject to liver damages. By CT scan, the liver is demonstrated with enlargement and plump margin. For those with complicating ascites, ultrasound demonstrates liquid dark area in the abdominal cavity. Some patients with coupled peritonitis is demonstrated with observable peritoneal thickening.

9.2 Typical Cases

Case 1

[Brief Case History]

An 8-year-old boy, a primary school student, complained of fever, cough and wheezing for 2 days. The boy began to experience irregular fever with no known causes 2 days ago, with a body temperature of up to 39 °C. Other symptoms include paroxysmal cough, expectoration of yellowish thick sputum in a small quantity, wheezing, shortness of breath, chest distress, dysphagia, occasional abdominal pain that aggravated when coughing and was more severe around the navel. By physical examination, body temperature 37.9 °C, heart rate 117/min, breathing rate 33/min, and blood pressure 105/60 mmHg; the lips no cyanosis; pharynx apparently congested, no follicular hyperplasia on the posterior pharyngeal wall, and no white spots; degree II enlargement of both tonsils; by auscultation, a small quantity of fine moist rales and wheezing in both lungs. At the age of 3 years, the patient experienced 2 episodes of asthma, which improved after treatment. His mother had a medical history of asthma. The patient reported a history of contact to patients with fever like symptoms. Throat swab by CDC showed the M gene of type A influenza virus positive, the NP gene of swine H1N1 influenza virus positive, and the HA gene of type A H1N1 influenza virus positive. Routine blood test revealed WBC count 6.69×10^9/L, GR% 78.1 %, LY% 12.7 %, MONO% 7 %, and HGB 118 g/L. Blood biochemistry showed AST 52.5U/L, CK 2022.5U/L, CK-MB 35.1U/L, and troponin 1.08 ng/ml; CD3+ T cell count 332/ul, CD4+ T cell count 173/ul, CD8+ T cell count 106/ul, and the ratio of CD4+/CD8+ 1.63. Blood gas analysis revealed pH 7.4, $PaCO_2$ 35.7 mmHg, PaO_2 109 mmHg, AB 21.6 mmo1/L, and BE -3.7 mmol/L.

[**Radiological demonstration**] Fig. 9.1.

[**Diagnosis**] Influenza A (H1N1) pneumonia.

[**Discussion**]

The early chest radiological signs in pediatric patients with influenza A (H1N1) pneumonia are non-characteristic, resembling to common lung infection. Influenza A (H1N1) pneumonia can be radiologically demonstrated as increased and thickened lung markings in both lungs as well as small patches of opacity. Along with the progression of the disease, the small patches of opacity may fuse into large flakes of opacity and/or ground glass like opacity.

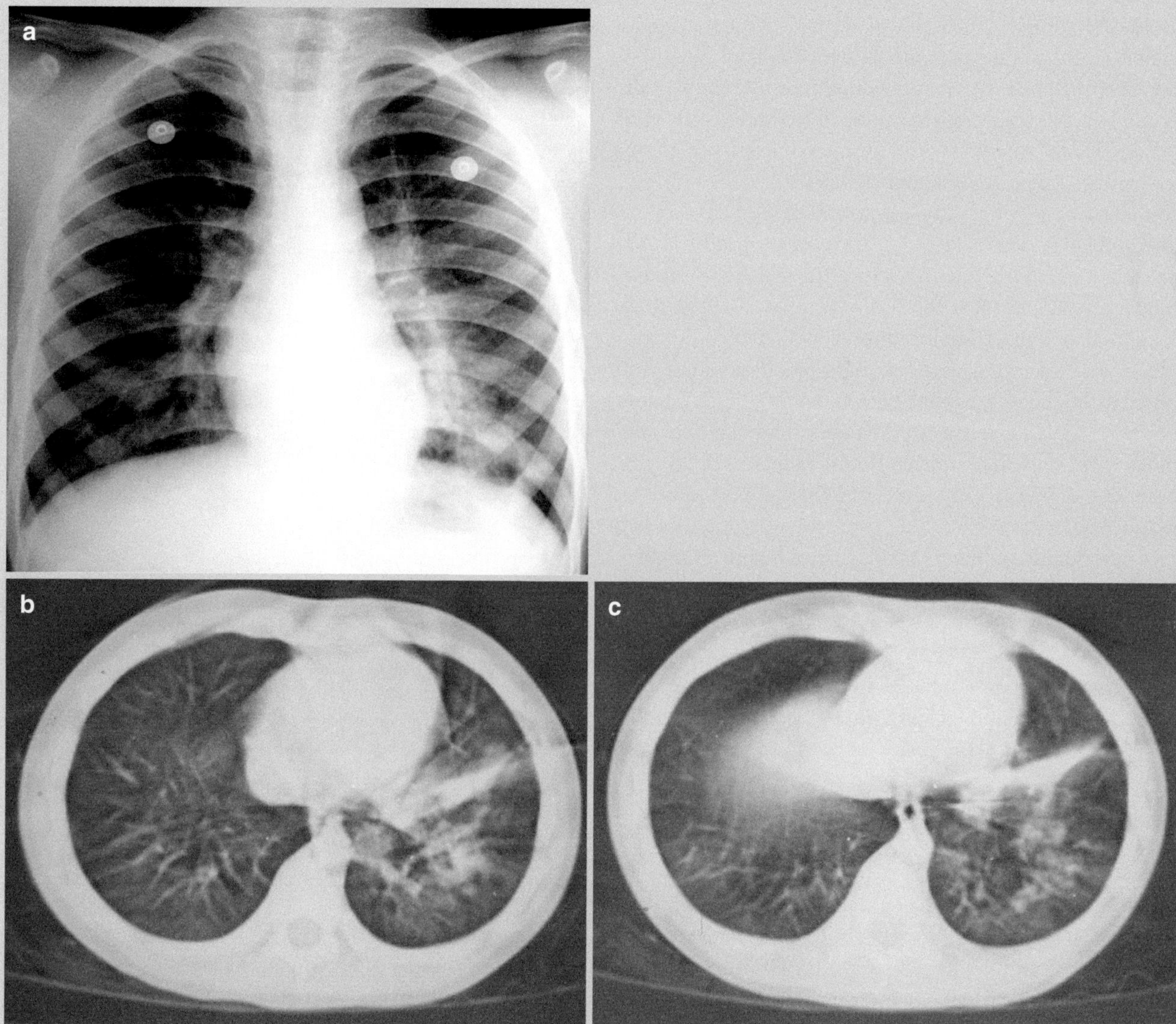

Fig. 9.1 Chest X-ray showed increased lung markings in both lungs, sporadic poorly defined patches of increased density opacity in the left middle and lower lung fields (**a**). CT scan demonstrated multiple consolidations, patches and GGO like opacities in the left lower lung lobe (**b**, **c**) (Reprint with permission from Hongjun Li and Ning Li (Eds), Radiology of Influenza A (H1N1), Springer, 2013)

Case 2

[**Brief Case History**]

A 4-years-old boy complained of fever and cough for 3 days. He experienced no chills, but poor appetite. By physical examination, bilateral lower lungs showed little moist rales. Chest X-ray and routine blood test immediately after onset showed no abnormality. Throat swab after hospitalization showed the M gene of type A influenza virus positive, the NP gene of swine H1N1 influenza virus positive, and the HA gene of type A H1N1 influenza virus positive.

[**Radiological demonstration**] Fig. 9.2

[**Diagnosis**] Pneumonia induced by type A H1N1 influenza virus.

[**Discussion**]

Radiologically, this case was shown with ground-glass opacity in bilateral lower lungs, which is consistent with the onset location of pneumonia induced by type A influenza. For this case, the symptoms are mild with early onset, which should be differentiated from other lung infections. Lobar pneumonia is demonstrated with consolidation of inflammatory lesion or lung segment. Lobular pneumonia is demonstrated with patchy opacity around bronchi. And the key point for its differentiation from pulmonary tuberculosis is the onset location, and the lower lungs are not the common onset location of pulmonary tuberculosis. For this case, its differential diagnosis from other pathogenic infections with interstitial inflammation is challenging, such as early mycoplasma pneumonia and other viral infections induced viral pneumonia. For this case, due to its early onset and mild symptoms, radiology helps little in the differential diagnosis. And this case is to raise awareness of the clinicians about the prevailing seasons of the disease. The possibility of pneumonia induced by type A influenza virus should be considered if relatively slight ground glass opacity is observed.

Early chest radiography shows no characteristic signs of pediatric pneumonia induced by type A H1N1 influenza virus. During its progressive stage, radiology demonstrates parenchymal lesions in lung, with parenchymal infiltration of singular or multiple small patches of opacity or their fusion into large opacity. In children, the progressive stage is shown with patchy opacity; while in infants, flakes and cotton like opacity.

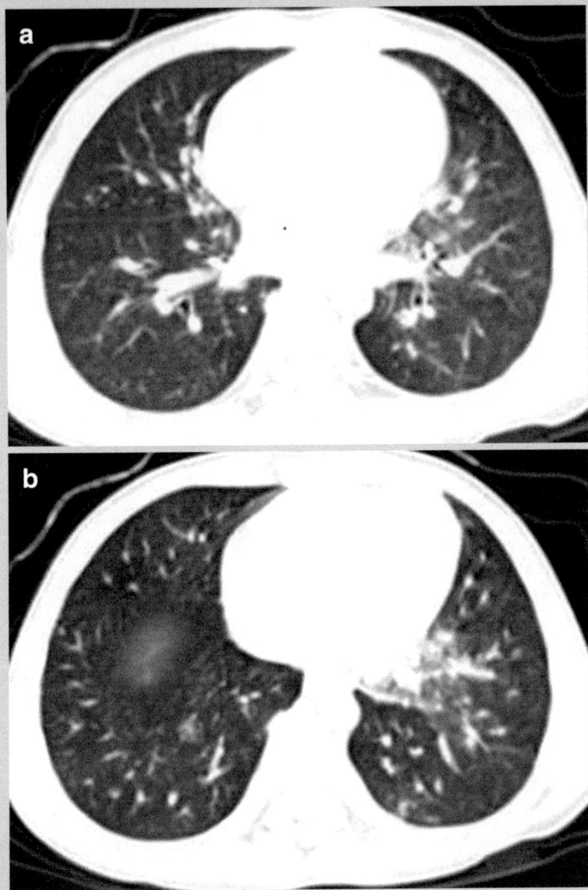

Fig. 9.2 (**a**, **b**) Chest CT scan revealed rare poorly defined ground glass opacity in bilateral lower lung lobes, which was predominantly in the left lower lung lobe

Case 3

[**Brief Case History**]

A 14-years-old boy complained of sore throat for 3 days; fever, fatigue and muscle soreness for 2 days. He experienced mild cough without sputum. By physical examination, body temperature 38.7 °C, pharyngeal congestion, and I degree tonsilar swelling. By routine blood test, WBC 4.97×10^9/L, and LY% 23.5 %. Chest CT scan on hospitalization showed the both lungs with multiple nodular and patchy high density opacity. Throat swab after hospitalization, the M gene of type A influenza virus was positive, the NP gene of swine H1N1 influenza virus positive, and the HA gene of type A H1N1 influenza virus positive.

[**Radiological demonstration**] Fig. 9.3

[**Diagnosis**] Pneumonia induced by type A H1N1 influenza virus.

[**Discussion**]

The early lesion of pneumonia induced by type A H1N1 influenza virus is an interstitial inflammation, which is mainly demonstrated as increased, thickened and blurred pulmonary vascular markings as well as grid like opacity and nodules in different degrees. For this case, the main radiological signs were multiple scattering nodular and patchy opacities, which should be differentiated from multiple pulmonary true nodules. The patients with multiple pulmonary metastatic nodules always have a medical history of primary disease. For this case, some of the inflammatory nodules disappeared after treatment, and the lesions in the right lower lung evoled into flake of high-density lesion.

The mild cases of pneumonia induced by type A H1N1 influenza virus show diversifying radiological signs, which are commonly non-specific. The radiological demonstrations include pulmonary parenchymal and interstitial inflammation, pleural inflammation, mediastinal and axillary lymphadenectasis, with lesions disseminating along bronchi, which resembles to viral pneumonia.

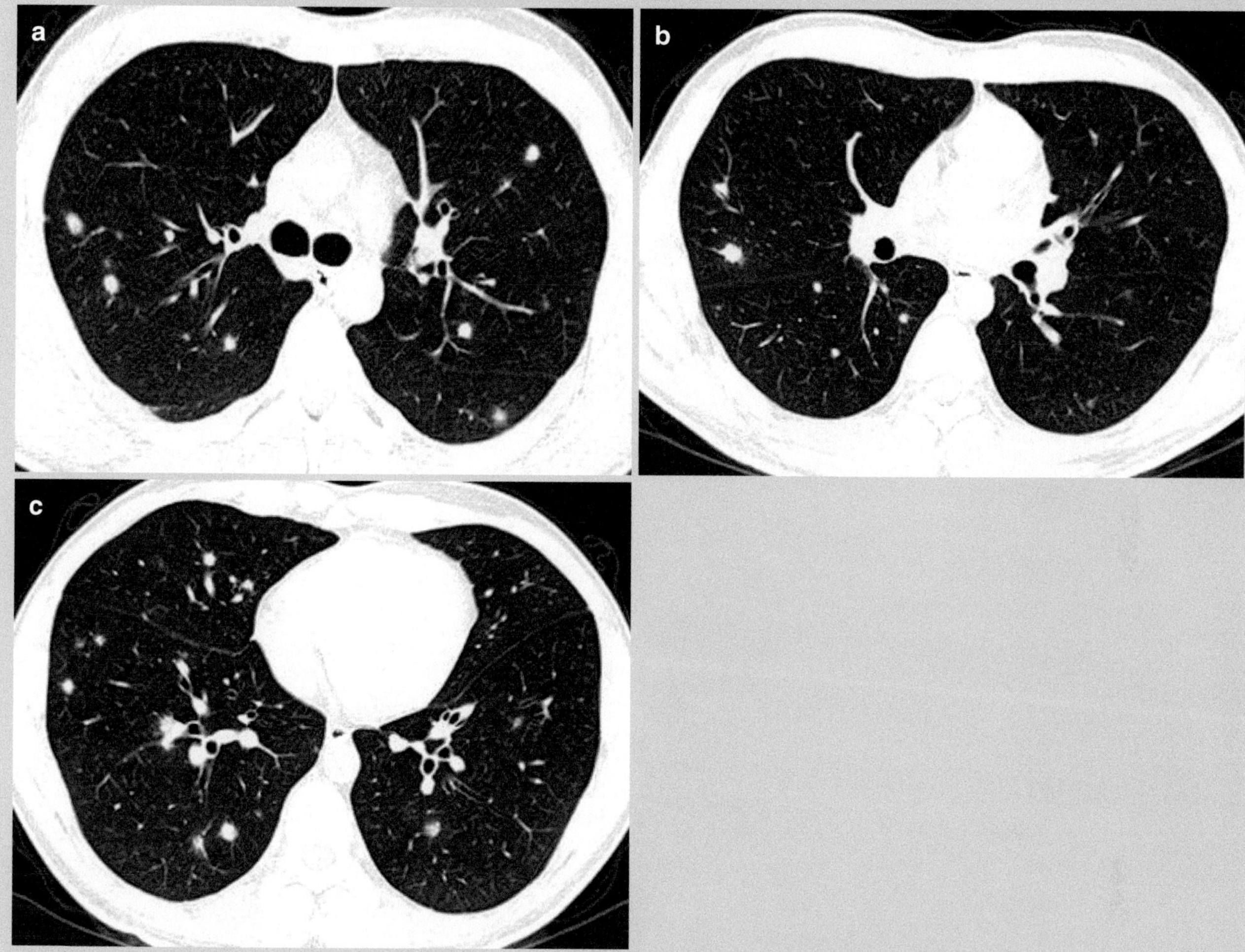

Fig. 9.3 (**a–c**) The both lungs were shown with multiple nodular and patchy high density opacity, predominantly in the right lower lung lobe

Case 4

[Brief Case History]

A 14-years-old girl was hospitalized due to chief complaints of fever and cough for 4 days. The patient experienced fever with no known cause on Nov. 6, 2009 with a body temperature of 37.5 °C. The fever was irregular with accompanying fatigue, paroxysmal cough, and expectoration of a small quantity yellowish sputum. Three days later, the patient experienced fever again with no known cause with a body temperature of 39.0 °C as well as aversion to cold, chest distress, dizziness, headache, systemic weakness, muscle soreness and other upsets. But the patient experienced no runny nose, no nasal obstruction, no chest pain, no shortness of breath, no palpitation, no hemoptysis, and no difficulty breathing. However, she had sore throat with sensation of foreign substance when swallowing and nausea. By physical examination, body temperature 37.3 °C, pulse 108/min, respiration 22/min, and blood pressure 102/63 mmHg. Lips showed no cyanosis; pharynx with obvious congestion, slight follicular hyperplasis at the posterior pharyngeal wall but no white spots, and both tonsils with II degree swelling. The both lungs showed coarse breathing sound as well as fine dry and moist rales. She reported a history of contact to a patient with similar fever and a history of contact to a patient with definitively diagnosed type A H1N1 influenza. In addition, her school was affected by type A H1N1 influenza. By CDC throat swab, the M gene of type A influenza virus was positive, the NP gene of swine H1N1 influenza virus positive, and the HA gene of type A H1N1 influenza virus positive. By routine blood test, WBC 15.31×10^9/L, GR% 82%, PLT 144.0×10^{12}/L, and HGB 140.9 g/L.

[**Radiological demonstration**] Fig. 9.4

[**Diagnosis**] Pneumonia induced by type A H1N1 influenza virus.

[**Discussion**]

Type A H1N1 influenza is more common in teenagers and young adults but rare in the elderly aged above 60 years. The patients commonly experience fever, cough, and sore throat; and some patients may also experience headache, nausea, vomiting, and diarrhea. Pneumonia is the most common complication of type A H1N1 influenza, which is radiologically demonstrated as lung parenchymal infiltration opacity. more commonly bilateral. The parenchymal infiltration is demonstrated as singular or multiple small patches of opacity or their fusion into large opacity and/or ground glass opacity. For this case, chest X-ray demonstrated multiple blurry flakes of opacity, while CT scan revealed multiple consolidations. Such findings indicated that CT scan should be timely ordered for clinical patients with respiratory symptoms in order to detect early lesions for appropriate treatment.

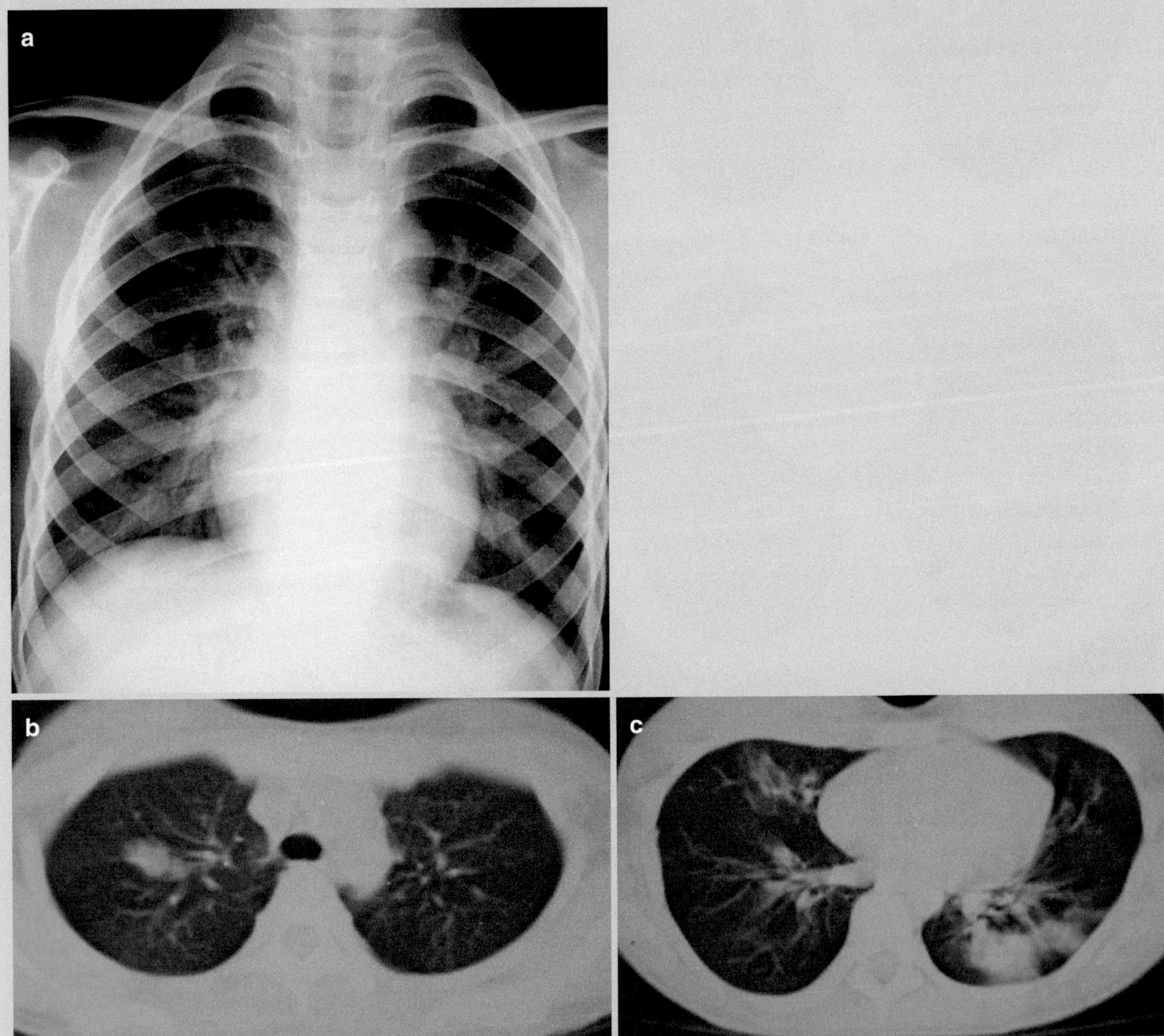

Fig. 9.4 Chest X-ray showed increased lung markings and multiple flakes of poorly defined opacity in both lungs (**a**); CT scan demonstrated multiple poorly defined consolidation opacity in the right upper lung lobe and the left lower lung lobe; and multiple cords like and patchy opacity in the right middle lung lobe (**b**, **c**) (Reprint with permission from Hongjun Li and Ning Li (Eds), Radiology of Influenza A (H1N1), Springer, 2013)

Case 5

[Brief Case History]

A 17-years-old teenager girl complained of fever and cough for 2 days with running nose but no aversion to cold, and malaise. She had a history of contact to a patient with type A influenza. By physical examination, body temperature 39.6 °C, pharyngeal congestion, and I degree tonsilar swelling. By throat swab, relevant items (such as FluA and SWH1) were shown positive.

[Radiological demonstration] Fig. 9.5.

[Diagnosis] Pneumonia induced by type A H1N1 influenza virus.

[Discussion]

In this case, CT scan showed focal ground-glass opacity and consolidation opacity with pleural effusion. The condition should be differentiated from bacterial pneumonia. Bacterial pneumonia is commonly demonstrated as lobar or segmental consolidation opacity that is confined and predominantly in one segment or one lobe. Its occurrence in both lungs or with diffuse lesion in one lung is rare, with slower progression of the leions than pneumonia induced by type A H1N1 influenza.

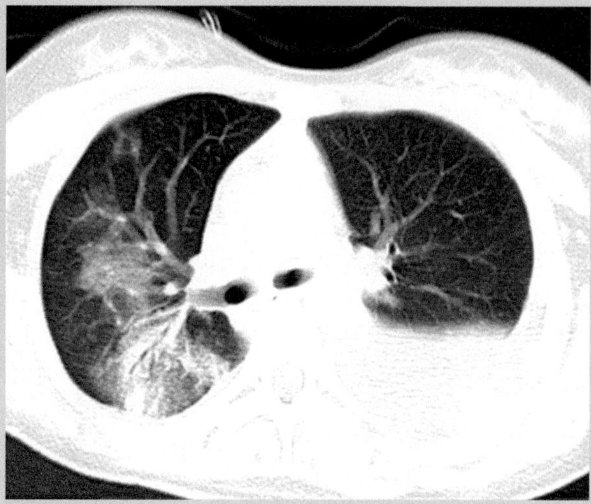

Fig. 9.5 Chest CT scan showed patchy high density opacity in the right middle and lower lung lobes, and left pleural effusion in a large quantity

Case 6

[Brief Case History]

A 5-years-old boy experienced fever, cough with expectoration, no aversion to cold or chills, systemic malaise, muscle soreness, and poor appetite. By physical examination, respiration 40/min, pulse 130/min, and body temperature 39 °C. The boy was conscious but low spirits, with dyspnea, nasal flaring, and a large quantity of rales in both lungs. He denied a history of contact to patient with type A influenza. Throat swab showed the M gene of type A influenza virus positive, the NP gene of swine H1N1 influenza virus positive, and the HA gene of type A H1N1 influenza virus positive. By routine blood test, WBC 1.9×10^9/L, GR% 69.9 %, and PLT 87×10^9/L. Blood chemistry revealed ALT 13.2U/L, AST 30.9/L, SpO_2 79-85 %.

[Radiological and pathological demonstrations] Fig. 9.6

[Diagnosis] Pneumonia induced by type A H1N1 influenza virus (severe case).

[Discussion]

Children are susceptible to type A H1N1 influenza, with high incidence and mortality. Being different from seasonal severe influenza that tends to affect the elderly aged above 65 years and young children aged under 2 years, 71 % of patients with severe pneumonia induced by type A H1N1 influenza virus are from the population aged 5–59 years. By chest X-ray, the lung lesions are characterized by early patches and flakes of high density opacity in local lung lobe or segment, and their rapid progression into large flakes and diffuse lesions, air bronchogram in multiple lobar or segmental consolidations, and compensatory emphysema in the contralateral non-diseased lung. In addition, the pulmonary parenchymal and interstitial lesions concur, with predominantly interstitial lesions in the advanced stage of the disease.

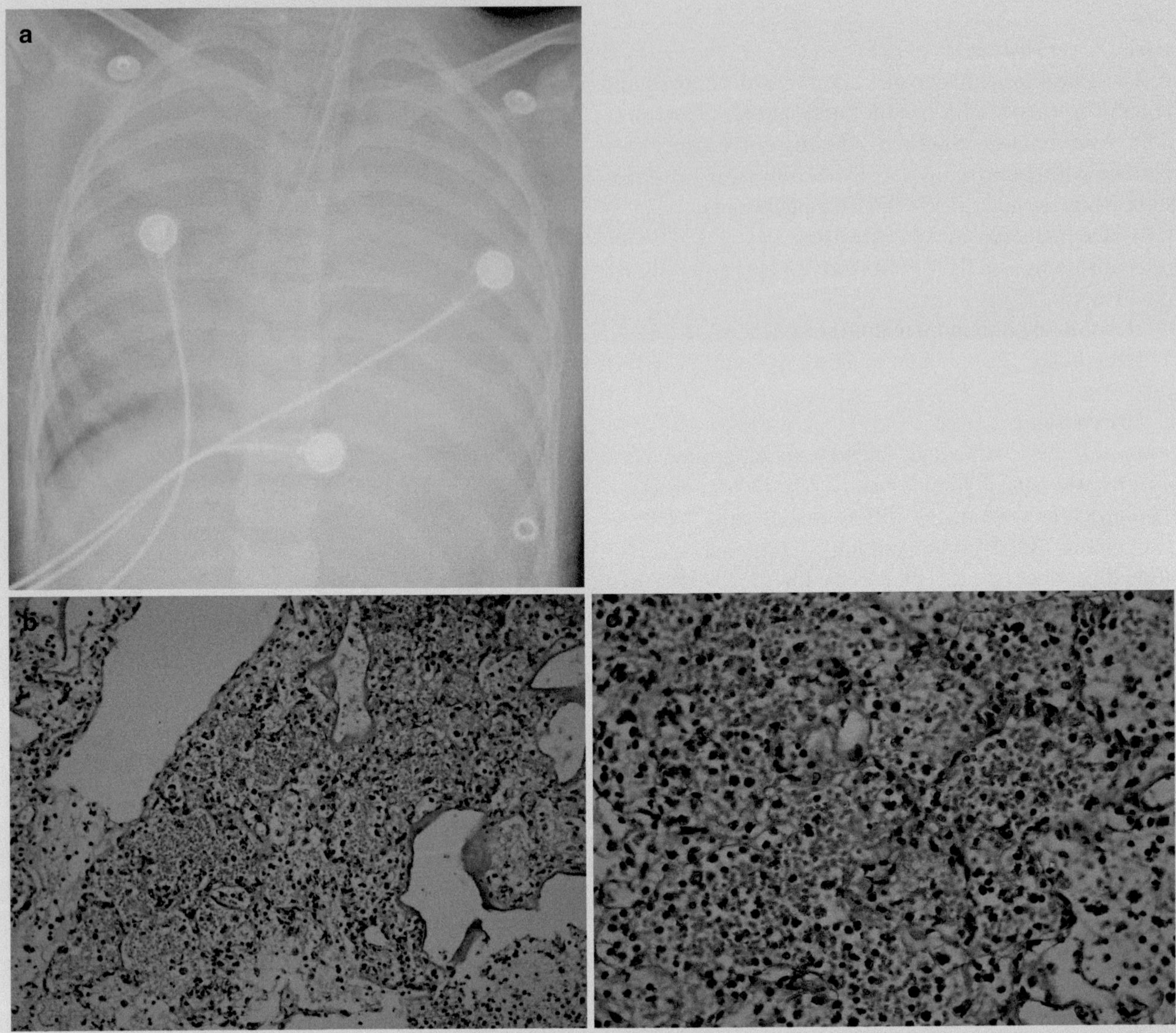

Fig. 9.6 Chest X-ray showed diffusely distributed high density opacity in both lungs that was predominantly in the left lung; poorly defined hila in both lungs; and poorly defined left diaphragm (**a**). Pathology demonstrated intra-alveolar hemorrhage and infiltration of inflammatory cells (**b**, **c**) (Reprint with permission from Hongjun Li and Ning Li (Eds), Radiology of Influenza A (H1N1), Springer, 2013)

Case 7

[Brief Case History]

A 29-years-old young woman experienced cough with no sputum and fever. Physical examination and laboratory test showed LDH 505U/L, post delivery, and a history of tonsilectomy.

[Radiological examination] Fig. 9.7

[Diagnosis] Pneumonia induced by type A H1N1 influenza virus.

[Discussion]

This case was radiologically demonstrated with multiple ground glass opacity and consolidation opacity in both lungs with some lesions closely adhering to the adjacent pleura, and the condition was clinically diagnosed as a severe case. And the clinical diagnosis was firstly considered to be pneumonia. For this case, the radiological signs are non-characteristic, and differential diagnosis from other factors induced pneumonia is necessary. But in this case, the symptoms occurred after delivery. Due to comparatively weak immunity during pregnancy, slight edema of respiratory mucosa tends to develop into respiratory infection. Pneumonia induced by type A H1N1 influenza virus in pregnancy is radiologically demonstrated as multiple ground glass opacity and consolidation opacity, with pleural lesion in some cases.

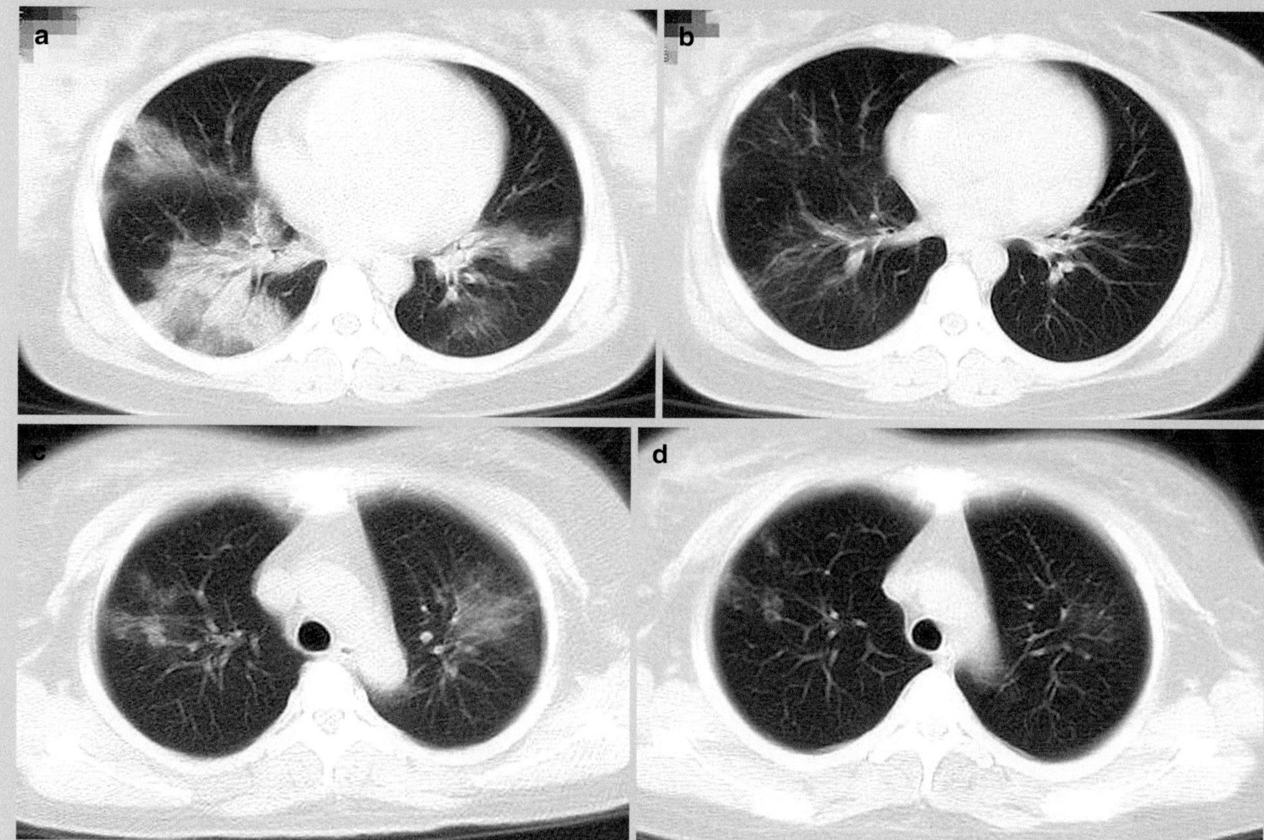

Fig. 9.7 Chest CT scan showed multiple patches and flakes of opacity in both lungs, some of which were ground-glass opacity and consolidation opacity (**a**, **b**). After treatment for 22 days and 30 days, CT scan showed absorption of the lesions (**c**, **d**)

Case 8

[Brief Case History]

A 31-years-old woman, 4 days after cesarean section, complained of fever, shortness of breath, and progressive dyspnea for 2 days. She began to cough 1 day ago with pinkish foam like sputum and show progressive dyspnea. Her condition failed to be improved by symptomatic therapy but aggravated. Physical examination showed a body temperature of 40 °C, and heart rate 136/min. The lips showed cyanosis, and breathing sound coarse with moist and dry rales all over the lungs. She reported a history of close contact to a patient with type A influenza. And throat swabs revealed the M gene of type A influenza virus negative, the NP gene of swine H1N1 influenza virus negative, and the HA gene of type A H1N1 influenza virus positive. Routine blood test showed WBC 12.97×10^9/L, GR% 91.1 %, RBC 3.24×10^{12}/L, and HGB 83 g/L.

[**Radiological demonstration**] Fig. 9.8

[**Diagnosis**] Pneumonia induced by type A H1N1 influenza virus.

[**Discussion**]

During pregnancy, the assistant total T cell count decreases and the activity of natural killer cells also decreases. As a result, the pregnant women are vulnerable to virus and fungal pneumonia. In mild cases, the lesions are demonsrated as ground glass opacity and small flakes of cotton like high density opacity in singular or multiple lung lobes. In severe cases, the lesions are demonstrated as masses of cotton like opacity, ground glass opacity, and air bronchogram in multiple lung lobes. Such lesions may progress within 24 h into diffuse high density opacity in both lungs with accompanying atelectasis, which may be complicated by unilateral or bilateral pleurisy, pleural effusion or pericardial effusion.

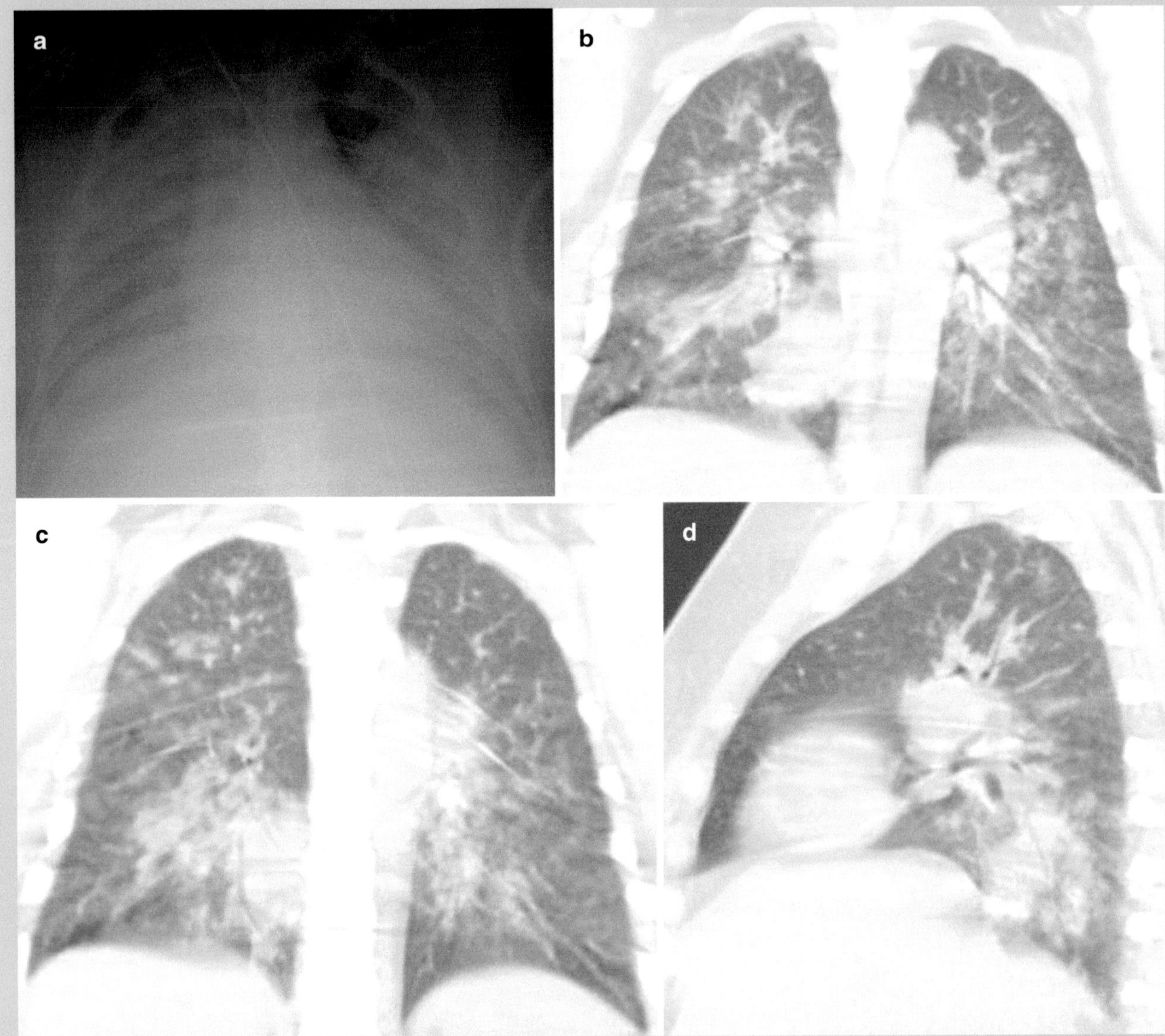

Fig. 9.8 Chest X-ray showed large flakes of high density opacity in both lungs that was predominantly in the right lung, and poorly defined hilum in both lungs (**a**). CT scan demonstrated multiple consolidation and ground glass opacity in both lungs, air bronchogram in the right upper lung lobe as well as thickened and deranged lung markings in both lungs (**b–f**) (Reprint with permission from Hongjun Li and Ning Li (Eds), Radiology of Influenza A (H1N1), Springer, 2013)

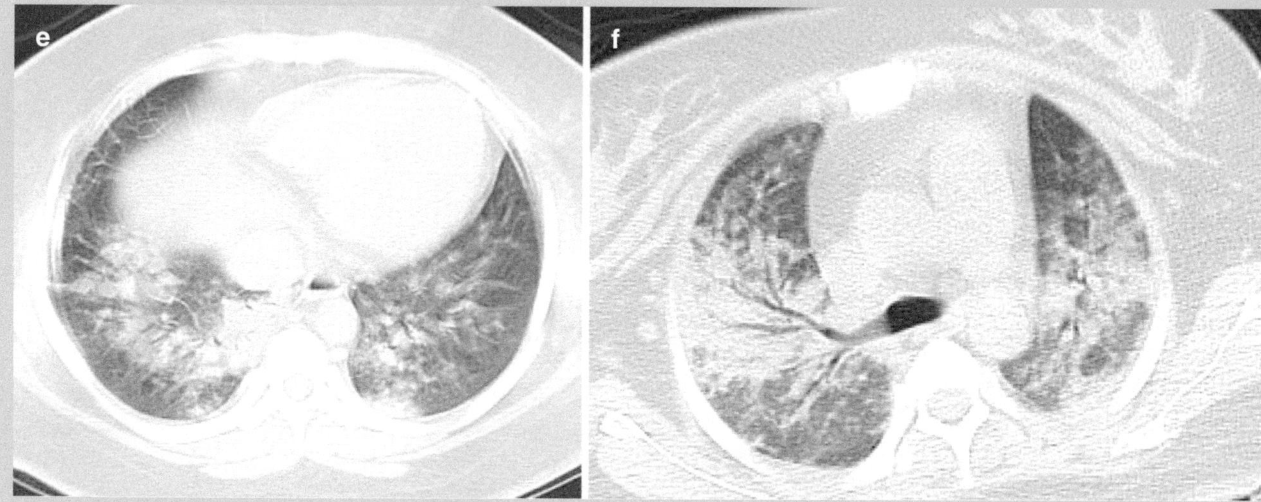

Fig. 9.8 (continued)

Case 9

[Brief Case History]

A 26-years-old young man experienced slight cough, expectoration of a little sputum, and fever with a body temperature of 38 °C. Laboratory test revealed WBC count 4.9×10^9/L, GR% 55.9 %, and LDH 135 U/L.

[Radiological demonstration] Fig. 9.9

[Diagnosis] Pneumonia induced by type A H1N1 influenza virus.

[Discussion]

In this case, the patient experienced symptoms of fever and slight cough, but CT scan showed local blurry lung markings in the left upper lung lobe and rare patches of ground glass opacity, which were small and confined. The diagnosis by radiology was considered to be lung inflammation.

In this case, the patient is a young man with rare and confined lesions in lungs by radiological examination. However, it still needs to be differentiated from bacterial and viral pneumonia, both of which may be local interstitial and parenchymal inflammation with lesions of confined ground glass opacity by radiology. The early manifestations of pneumonia induced by type A H1N1 influenza virus resemble to pneumonia induced by other viruses. Some previous studies were performed to stage slight, moderate and severe pneumonia induced by type A H1N1 influenza virus based on the radiological findings. Some studies have demonstrated that chest ultrasound in the emergency room can detect interstitial lesions of early pneumonia induced by type A H1N1 influenza virus, while CR fails to detect any lung lesion during the same stage of the disease. However, these studies also indicated that CT scan can more favorably show the lung lesions for the patients with pneumonia induced by type A H1N1 influenza virus, especially during the early stage and for the severe cases.

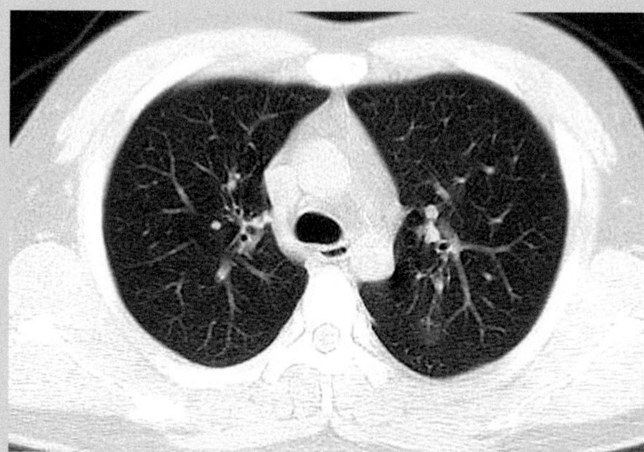

Fig. 9.9 CT scan showed small flakes of ground glass opacity near the oblique fissure in the left upper lung lobe

Case 10

[Brief Case History]

A 43-years-old woman complained of fever and dry cough.

[Radiological demonstration] Fig. 9.10

[Diagnosis] Pneumonia induced by type A H1N1 influenza virus.

[Discussion]

Radiologically, the patient showed subpleural patchy opacity with lobular distribution in sizes of 1–1.5 cm, with multiple lung lobes involved. As a result, lung inflammation was considered and differentiation is needed to define the diagnosis from bacterial pneumonia, fungal pneumonia, Pneumocystis jiroveci pneumonia and other viral pneumonia. Pneumonia caused by bacteria (commonly staphylococcus, pneumonic diplococcus and streptococcus) is pathologically characterized by bronchitis, peribronchitis, alveolitis, peri-alveolitis and multiple lobular pneumonia. And it is radiologically demonstrated as thickened lung marking as well as patchy and nodular opacity that are commonly located in the medial lung and fuse within 2–3 days. Pneumonia caused by fungi (commonly aspergillus and cryptococcus) is pathologically characterized by exudative and purulent inflammation in lungs. And it is radiologically demonstrated as singular or multiple nodules, lumps or cavities. Pneumonia caused by Pneumocystis jiroveci is pathologically characterized by serous and exudative alveolitis. And it is radiologically demonstrated as lobar or segmental lesions, which are poorly defined patchy opacity along bronchi commonly in bilateral middle and lower lung fields. In some cases, the lesions may show progression and fusion within several hours or several days. Pneumonia caused by other viruses, such as adenovirus, respiratory syncytial virus, measles virus and cytomegalovirus, commonly occurs in young children, which is pathologically characterized by bronchitis and bronchopneumonia with infiltration of inflammatory cells that are predominantly mononuclear cells. And it is radiologically demonstrated as small nodular opacity and patchy opacity that are commonly located in middle and medial parts of bilateral middle and lower lung fields.

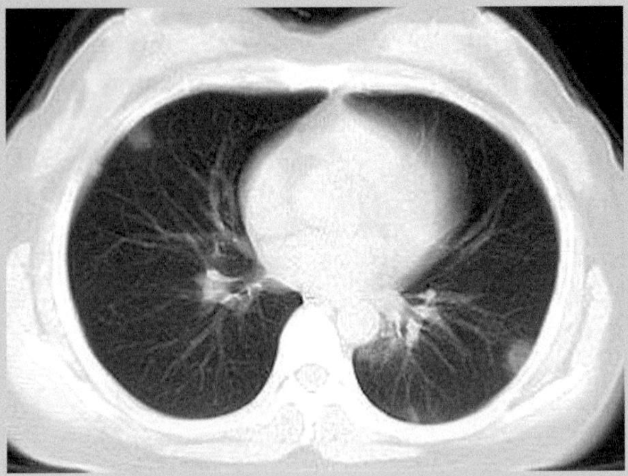

Fig. 9.10 CT scan showed subpleural patchy opacity in the right middle lung lobe and the left lower lung lobe

Case 11

[Brief Case History]

A 52-year-old man complained of cough, expectoration of a little sputum, and fever. Laboratory test revealed WBC count 6.5×10^9/L, GR% 85.5 % and LDH 160U/L.

[Radiological demonstration] Fig. 9.11

[Diagnosis] Pneumonia induced by type A H1N1 influenza virus.

[Discussion]

Radiologically, this case is demonstrated with multiple patchy opacities along bronchovascular bundles with varying density in both lungs, some of which were shown to be ground-glass opacity and blurry small nodular opacity. Lung inflammation should be firstly considered for diagnosis. Pneumonia induced by type A H1N1 influenza virus is radiologically demonstrated as flakes and patches consolidations and ground glass opacity, with predominant lobular distribution.

Pneumonia induced by type A H1N1 influenza virus should be differentiated from bacterial pneumonia, Pneumocystis jiroveci pneumonia and other viral pneumonia. For this case, its differential diagnosis from bacterial pneumonia is challenging. Bacterial pneumonia is radiologically demonstrated as thickened lung markings and more obvious lobar and segmental distribution. The lesions of pneumonia induced by type A H1N1 influenza virus are distributed in multi-lobes and segments with low density. The lesions of bacterial pneumonia integrate or show morphological changes within 2–3 days. Pneumonia caused by fungi and Pneumocystis jiroveci is pathologically alveolitis and is radiologically demonstrated as singular or multiple nodules, lumps or cavities, otherwise, lobar and segmental lesions as well as blurry patchy opacity commonly bilateral middle and lower lung fields along bronchi. Pneumonia caused by other virus is radiologically demonstrated as small nodular opacity and patchy opacity that are commonly located in middle and medial parts of bilateral middle and lower lung fields.

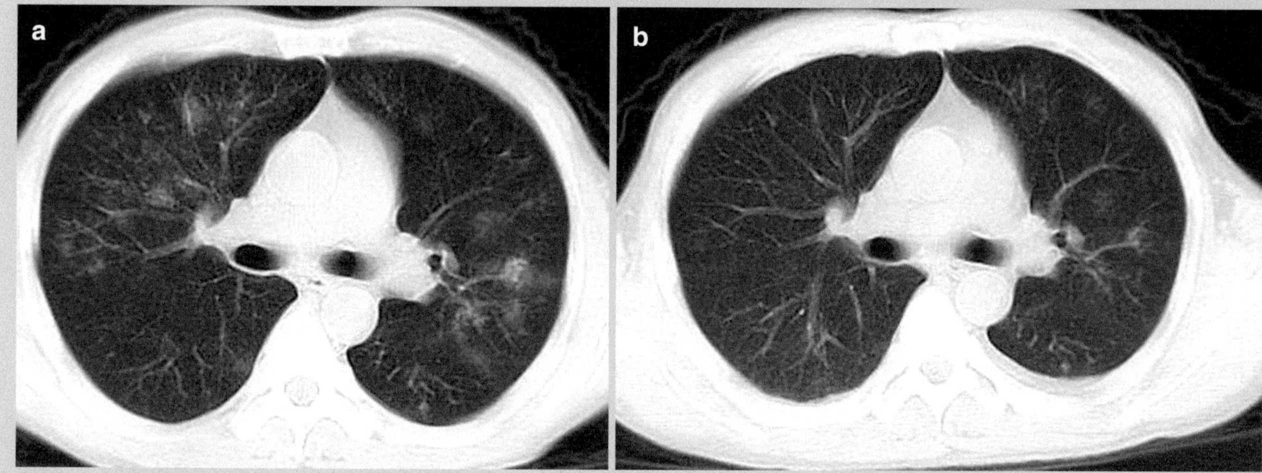

Fig. 9.11 CT scan showed multiple small nodules and blurry patchy opacity distributing along lung markings in both lungs (**a**). Reexamination by CT scan after treatment for 10 days showed decreased lesions, indicating absorption (**b**)

Case 12

[Brief Case History]

A 41-year-old man complained of high fever, wheezing and progressive dyspnea for 5 days. He had taken cephalosporin by himself, with no obvious improvement. And 2 days ago, he began to cough up pinkish foamy sputum. The patient reported a history of contact to a patient with type A influenza. By routine blood test 3 days ago, WBC count 12.11×10^9/L. And routine blood test on admission showed WBC count 17.45×10^9/L, and GR% 81.1 %. Chest X-ray in another hospital revealed inflammation in both lungs, and predominantly in the left lower lung lobe. By throat swab after being hospitalized, the M gene of type A influenza virus positive, the NP gene of swine H1N1 influenza virus positive, and the HA gene of type A H1N1 influenza virus positive. Sputum smear revealed cocci positive.

[Radiological demonstration] Fig. 9.12

[Diagnosis] Pneumonia induced by type A H1N1 influenza virus.

[Discussion]

For this case, CT scan demonstrated patchy opacity and ground glass opacity at lung margin of both lungs, which is consistent to the early radiological sign of pneumonia induced by type A influenza virus. The lesions were predominantly located in the left lower lung lobe. In this case, routine blood test indicated increased WBC count, which continued to increase after hospitalization. Sputum smear revealed cocci positive, indicating bacterial infection that complicated primary viral infection.

For this case, it should be differentiated from simplex bacterial pneumonia, which is commonly demonstrated as lobar or segmental high density opacity that is comparatively confined and is not predominantly located at lung margin. This case also needs to be differentiated from mycoplasmal pneumonia, which is radiologically demonstrated as centrilobular ground glass opacity or consolidation, which may develop into segmental or lobar consolidation and is commonly fan like in shape. Such radiological signs are rarely found in the cases of pneumonia induced by type A influenza virus.

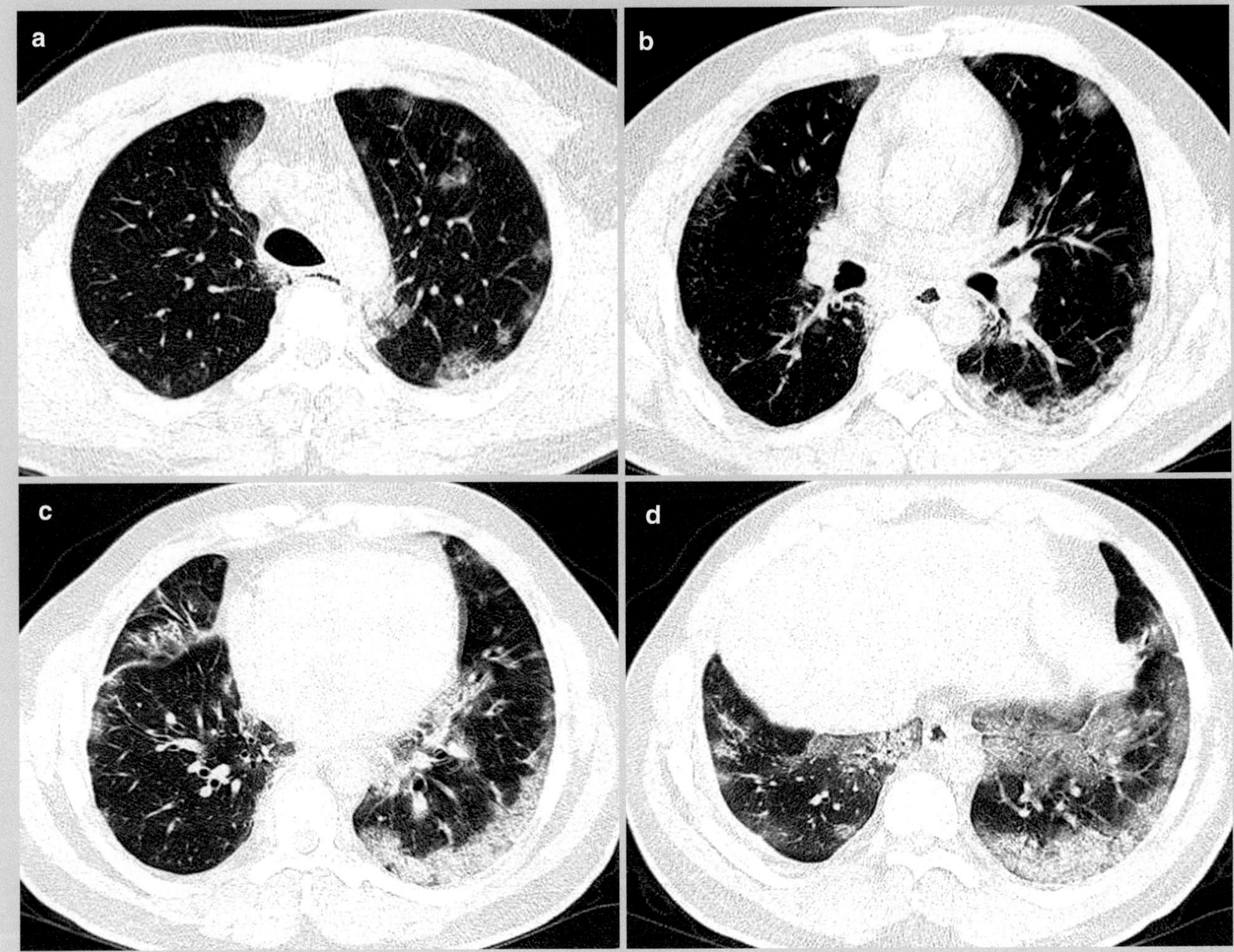

Fig. 9.12 Chest CT scan showed multiple flakes and cords like high density opacity and ground glass opacity in both lungs that was predominantly in the left lower lung lobe. The lesions were revealed to be commonly located at the lung margin (**a–d**)

Case 13

[Brief Case History]

A 54-year-old woman complained of cough, expectoration of whitish yellow sputum, and fever. She reported medical history of hypertension and diabetes. Laboratory test revealed LDH 383U/L.

[**Radiological demonstration**] Fig. 9.13

[**Diagnosis**] Pneumonia induced by type A H1N1 influenza virus.

[**Discussion**]

The patient was radiologically revealed with multiple patchy/flaky consolidations in both lungs, which closely adhered to the adjacent pleura, and pneumonia should be firstly considered for clinical diagnosis. The patient had a medical history of diabetes and was vulnerable to viral and/or bacterial infection.

Radiologically, differential diagnosis should be made from bacterial pneumonia, fungal pneumonia, Pneumocystis jiroveci pneumonia and other viral pneumonia. Pneumonia induced by type A H1N1 influenza virus is radiologically demonstrated as ground glass opacity, possibly consolidation opacity and centrilobular nodular opacity, and accompanying pleural response. The lesions of severe pneumonia induced by type A influenza virus are pathologically revealed as diffuse alveolar damage. And chest CT scan shows severe pneumonia induced by type A influenza virus with diversifying lesions, with no definitive specificity. Both lungs are shown to be involved with multiple flakes of ground glass opacity as well as consolidation and nodules that are more commonly located in the bilateral peripheral middle and lower lung lobes. In this case, more consolidations were revealed, which may be related to the underlying disease of diabetes. After appropriate therapy was given, the lesions were shown to be obviously absorbed.

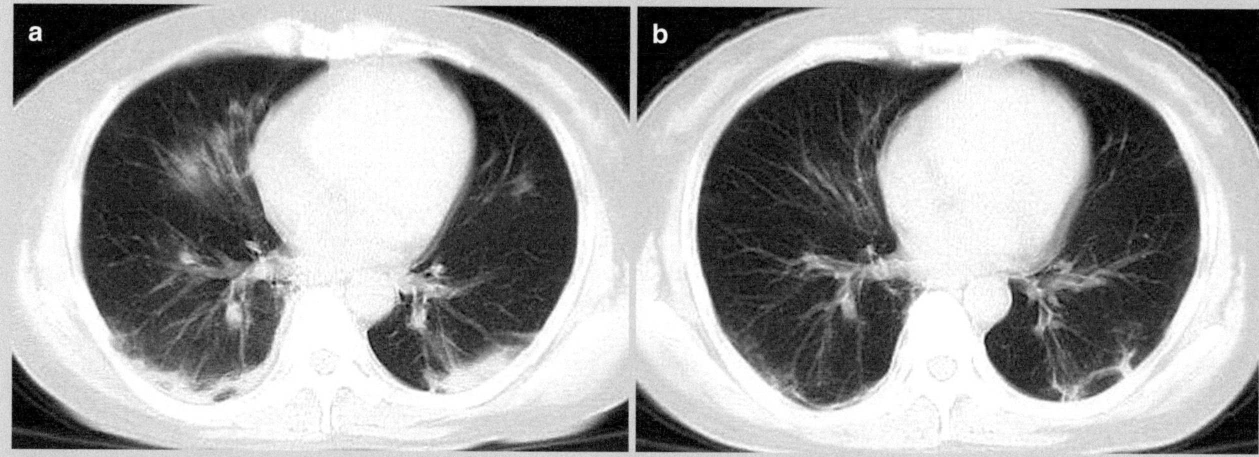

Fig. 9.13 CT scan showed patchy and curved flake like opacity in the right middle lung lobe, lingular segment of the left lung, and subpleural areas in bilateral lower lung lobes, some of which were dense (**a**). Reexamination after treatment for 9 days showed absorption of the lesions and residual curved linear opacity in subpleural areas (**b**)

Case 14

[**Brief Case History**]

A 58-year-old man complained of slight cough, expectoration of whitish thick sputum, and fever. Laboratory test revealed WBC count 9.7×10^9/L, GR% 92.8 %, and LDH 427U/L. He experienced respiratory failure of degree I.

[**Radiological demonstration**] Fig. 9.14

[**Diagnosis**] Pneumonia induced by type A H1N1 influenza virus.

[**Discussion**]

The patient was radiologically showed with multiple flakes of ground glass opacity in upper and lower lobes of both lungs that were multiple and closely adhered to the adjacent pleura. Pneumonia should be firstly considered for clinical diagnosis. Pneumonia induced by type A H1N1 influenza virus is commonly demonstrated as unilateral or bilateral diffuse or multiple patches of ground glass opacity with or with no consolidation that is mostly located around bronchovascular bundles or in the subpleural area. However, such radiological signs are non-specific, and differential diagnosis should be made from Pneumocystis jiroveci pneumonia, other viral pneumonia, and mycoplasmal pneumonia. Pneumonia caused by Pneumocystis jiroveci is pathologically characterized by serous and exudative alveolitis. And it is radiologically demonstrated as lobar or segmental ground glass opacity. In some cases, the lesions may show progression and fusion within several hours or several days. Pneumonia caused by other virus is radiologically demonstrated as patches/flakes of ground glass opacity with/without consolidation, no mediastinal lymphadenectasis, and rarely pleural effusion. Compared to pneumonia caused by type A H1N1 influenza virus, other viral pneumonia shows more lesions of minor airways, which are demonstrated as centrilobular nodules that are more common in young children. And other viral pneumonia is pathologically characterized by bronchitis and bronchopneumonia with infiltration of inflammatory cells that are predominantly mononuclear cells. In addition, it is radiologically demonstrated as small nodular opacity and patchy opacity that are commonly located in middle and medial parts of bilateral middle and lower lung fields. Mycoplasmal pneumonia is radiologically demonstrated as ground glass opacities with/without consolidation and sporadic small nodules. Compared to pneumonia caused by type A H1N1 influenza virus, mycoplasmal pneumonia commonly involves one lung, with mediastinal lymphadenectasis and pleural effusion.

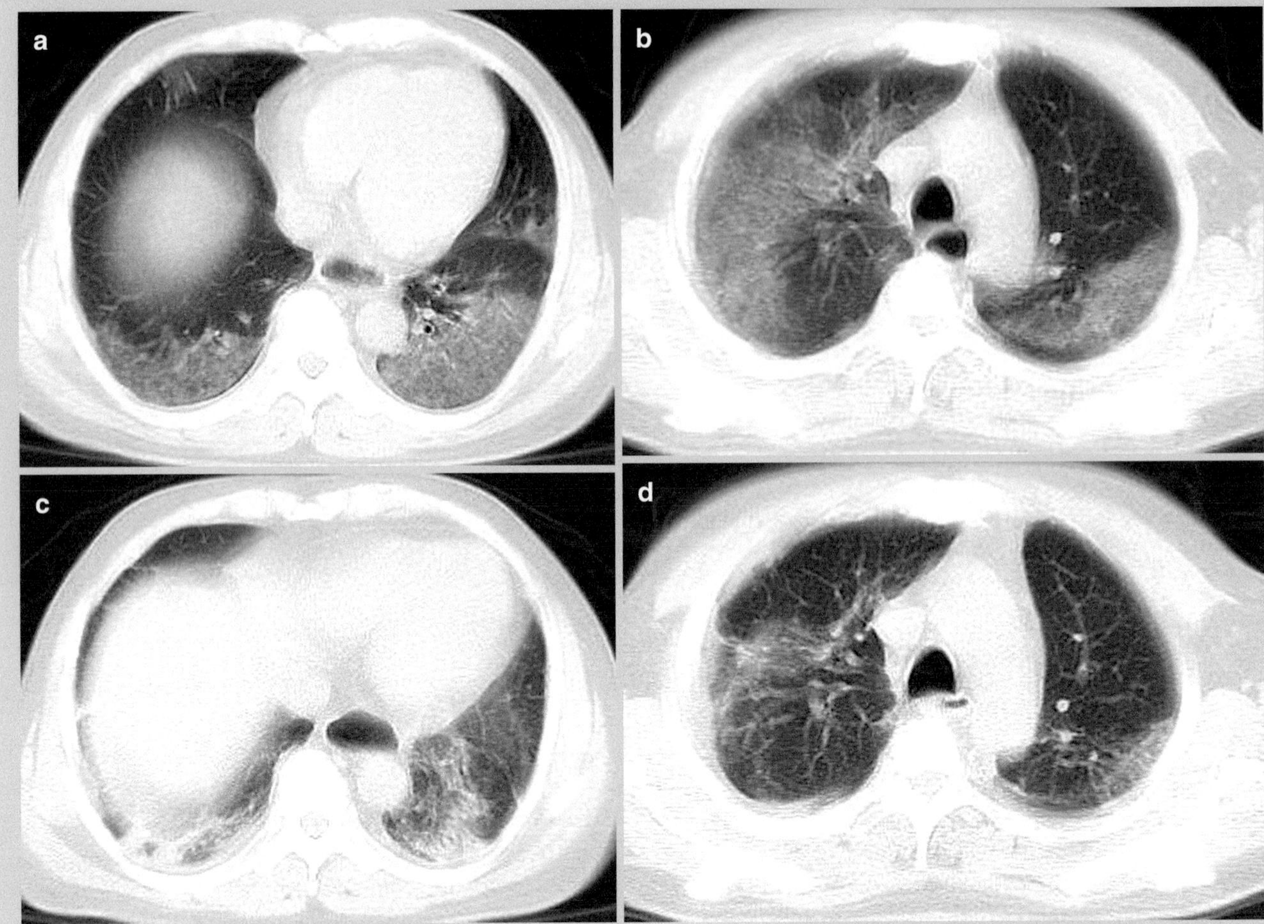

Fig. 9.14 CT scan showed multiple flakes of ground glass opacity in both lungs that closely adhered to the pleura (**a**, **b**). Reexaminations after treatment for 27 days (**c**) and 36 days (**d**), the lesions were shown with absorption. But curved linear or strips and flakes of opacity was revealed, with local pleural thickening

Case 15

[**Brief Case History**]

A 38-year-old man complained of cough rarely with sputum and fever. Laboratory test revealed WBC count 9.2×10^9/L, GR% 69.6 %, and LDH 182U/L.

[**Radiological demonstration**] Fig. 9.15

[**Diagnosis**] Pneumonia induced by type A H1N1 influenza virus.

[**Discussion**]

The patient was radiologically showed with flakes of ground glass opacity in the right upper lung lobe, with thick-wall cavity inside and partly with consolidation. Pneumonia should be firstly considered for clinical diagnosis. In literature reports, pneumonia induced by type A H1N1 influenza virus is rarely reported with lesions of cavity, and this case is categorized into a rare case. The cavity might be one of the radiological signs of pneumonia induced by type A H1N1 influenza virus itself, and may also be a radiological sign of the complication. And it should be differentiated from bacterial pneumonia and fungal pneumonia. Pneumonia caused by bacteria may show cavity during its progression, which is commonly found in the cases of streptococcal and gram-negative bacterial infections. Clinically, pus or sputum with unpleasant odor is common, and the cavity is commonly revealed in consolidation opacity with poorly defined bounary and sometimes with air-fluid level. Pneumonia caused by fungi is radiologically demonstrated as singular or multiple nodules, lumps or cavities. Typical pneumocystis pneumonia is radiologically demonstrated as thin-wall cavity with no or rare surrounding lesions. Aspergillosis is radiologically demonstrated as cavity in poorly defined flakes of consolidation opacity with varying thickness of the wall. The typical cases are shown with nodules or lumps in the cavity and observable gas containing crescent sign, and aspergilloma is mobile along with posture changes. Pneumonia caused by Pneumocystis jiroveci, if complicated by bacterial or fungal infection, is radiologically demonstrated as cavities or cavities in lobar or segmental consolidation.

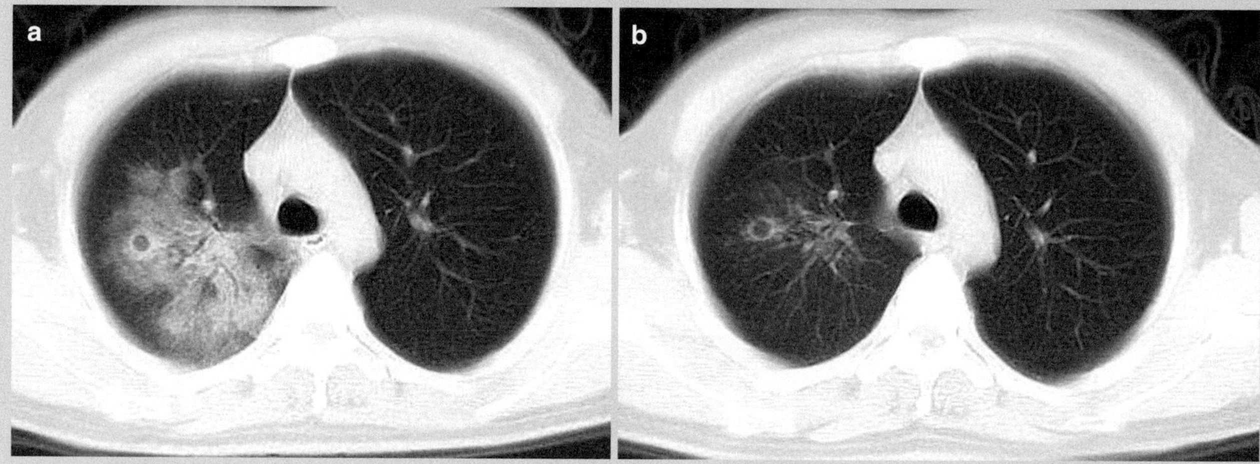

Fig. 9.15 CT scan showed flakes of poorly defined opacity in the right upper lung lobe, with bronchi sign and thick-wall translucent opacity (**a**); Reexamination after treatment showed thin-wall translucent opacity (**b**)

Case 16

[Brief Case History]

A 37-year-old man complained of cough, expectoration, and a sore throat for 7 days. He experienced expectoration of whitish foamy sputum and a fever for 4 days with the highest body temperature of 39 °C. Other symptoms included aversion to cold, wheezing and difficulty breathing for 2 days. By physical examination, the pharynx was shown with obvious congestion, and the right tonsil swollen in degree I. Both lungs were found with moist rales. By routine blood test, WBC count 8.9×10^9/L, GR% 55 %, and LY% 34 %. By throat swab after hospitalization, the M gene of type A influenza virus positive, the NP gene of swine H1N1 influenza virus positive, and the HA gene of type A H1N1 influenza virus negative.

[Radiological demonstration] Fig. 9.16

[Diagnosis] Pneumonia induced by type A influenza virus.

[Discussion]

Early pneumonia induced by type A H1N1 influenza virus is radiologically demonstrated as roughly symmetrical ground glass opacity in both lungs. Initially, the virus mainly invades the lung interstitium and the early lesions are mainly changes of interstitial pneumonia, which are radiologically demonstrated as multiple ground glass density opacity in both lungs. Further progression of the lesions causes alveolar exudation or secondary bacterial/fungal infection, which is shown as consolidation of lungs tissue. The consolidation opacity is commonly located at the lung margin, with fusion of some lesions and air bronchogram. The progression of lesions may also cause fibrosis of lung tissue, which is radiologically demonstrated as widened interlobular sepum and honeycomb like opacity in one or both lungs.

For this case, it needs to be differentiated from other viral pneumonia, such as SARS. Both are viral inflammation, with extremely similar radiological signs during their early stage. The early radiological signs include fibrin exudation, consolidation, and their further progression into pulmonary fibrosis. Severe pneumonia caused by type A influenza virus is radiologically demonstrated as flakes of exudation and fusion as well as reticular or nodular high density opacity in both lungs that fuse into poorly defined cloudy opacity. And the lesions may further develop into extensive consolidation opacity, which needs to differentiate from consolidation of lung tissue in the cases of lobar pneumonia. In combination to the case history and the illness course, the differential diagnosis can be made.

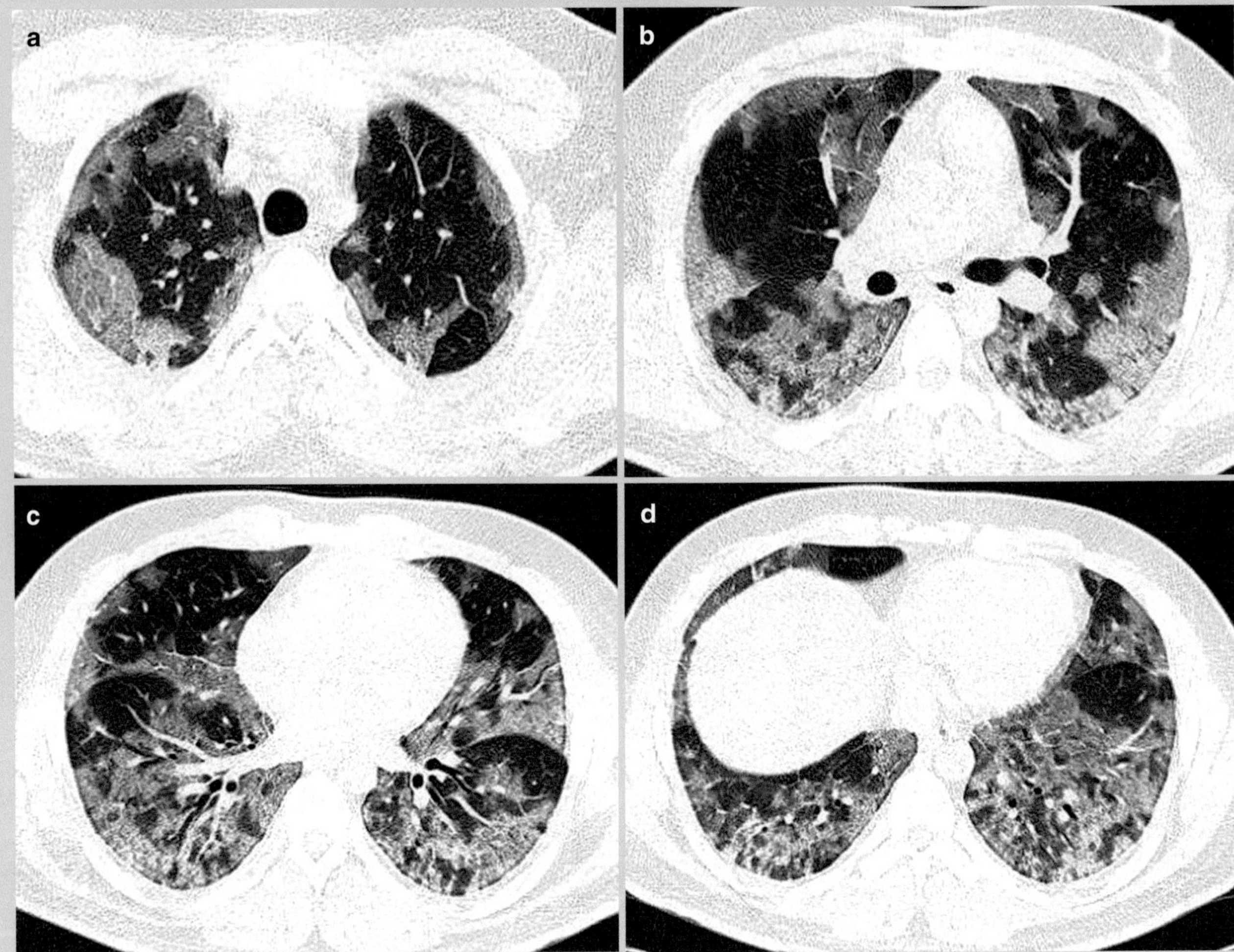

Fig. 9.16 CT scan showed sporadic flakes of high density opacity and ground glass opacity that were predominantly in bilateral lower lungs lobes as well as consolidation of partial lung tissues with gas containing bronchi (**a–d**)

Case 17

[**Brief Case History**]

A 41-year-old man experienced fever and cough for 10 days with accompanying sore throat, systemic malaise, and muscle soreness. He began to experience high fever 5 days ago with the highest body temperature of 39.6 °C. Chest X-ray in another hospital showed inflammation in both lungs. After intravenous infusion of cephalosporin, the symptom of fever was slightly improved. Recently, the patient began to experience symptoms of orthopnea and bloody sputum. By physical examination, the pharynx congested, and the bilateral tonsils swollen in degree I. Moist rales in both lungs, predominantly in lower lungs. By routine blood test on admission, WBC count 10.6×10^9/L, and LY% 7.5 %. Sputum smear revealed cocci positive and bacillus negative. By throat swab after hospitalization, the M gene of type A influenza virus positive, the NP gene of swine H1N1 influenza virus positive, and the HA gene of type A H1N1 influenza virus negative.

[**Radiological demonstration**] Fig. 9.17.

[**Diagnosis**] Influenza A (H1N1) pneumonia; Subcutaneous emphysema in the left thoracic wall.

[**Discussion**]

In this case, lung consolidation opacities were predominantly located in the left lower lung lobe a long period of development. Ground glass opacities sporadically distributed in both lungs, indicating virus infection. After treatment by anti-inflammatory therapy, his condition was improved, indicating a complication of bacterial infection. The patient experienced respiratory failure and was given several times of CPR, which resulted in ribs fracture and subcutaneous emphysema of the chest wall. The key point for differential diagnosis from lobar pneumonia is that the lesion of consolidation in the cases of lobar pneumonia is located within one lung lobe or one lung segment. However, in this case, the lesion of consolidation was concurrent with sporadic GGO in the left lower lung. Therefore, their differential diagnosis can be made in combination to clinical manifestations and the absorption stage of lobar pneumonia.

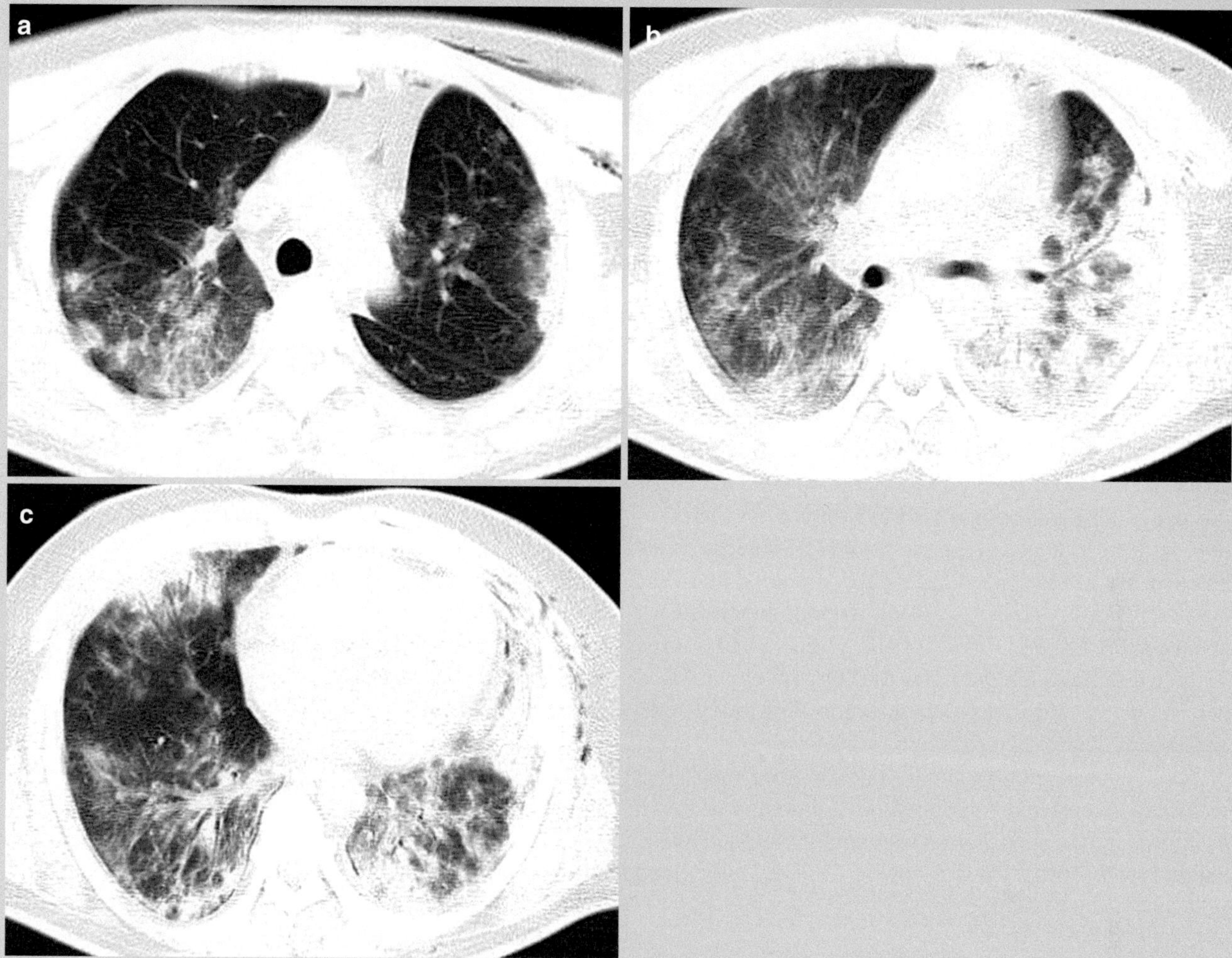

Fig. 9.17 Chest CT scan showed sporadic flakes of high density opacity and ground glass opacity, predominantly in bilateral lower lung lobes; consolidation of partial lung tissues in the left lower lung lobe; beads like air density opacity in the left thoracic wall (**a–c**)

Case 18

[**Brief Case History**]

A 54-year-old man complained of fever for 7 days, cough and expectoration for 6 days, as well as difficulty breathing for 2 days which aggravated during nights. He denied a history of contact to patient with type A influenza. And his physical signs included throat congested, no tonsil swollen, and moist rales in both lungs. Laboratory throat swab test showed etiological factors related to influenza A (H1N1), including FluA and SWH1, positive.

[**Radiological demonstration**] Fig. 9.18.

[**Diagnosis**] Pneumonia induced by type A H1N1 influenza virus.

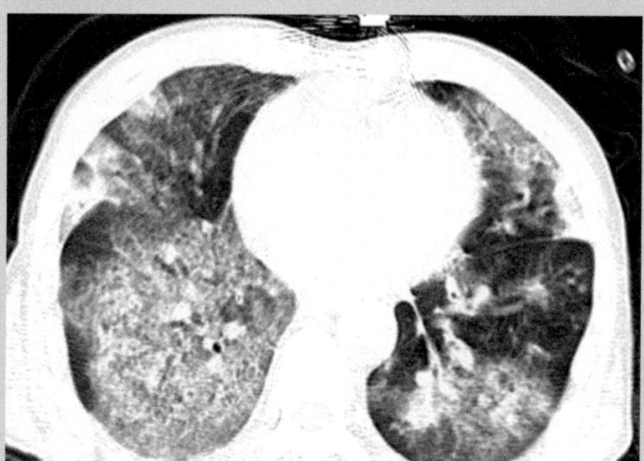

Fig. 9.18 Chest CT scan showed ground glass opacity and patches of high density opacity in both lungs, with local consolidations

[Discussion]

In this case, the lesions were diffusely distributed in the right lower lung field, accompanied by interstitial thickening. And the condition should be differentiated from SARS. The early manifestations of pneumonia induced by type A H1N1 influenza virus resemble to SARS, demonstrated as fibrinous exudation and consolidation that further progress into pulmonary interstitial fibrosis. Severe and critical pneumonia induced by type A H1N1 influenza virus are demonstrated as flakes of alveolar exudation with fusion, network like or nodular opacity and inflammatory consolidation in both lungs, rarely with pleural effusion. The lesions are commonly located in both lower lungs, which are radiologically demonstrated as large flakes of dense consolidation opacity along with their progression.

Case 19

[Brief Case History]

A 42-year-old man complaint of fever and cough for 5 days. By physical examination, body temperature 39.5 °C, the tonsils swollen in degree I, and the breathing sound of both lungs coarse. He reported a non-definitive history of contact to patient with type A influenza. By laboratory throat swab, the M gene of type A H1N1 influenza virus positive, the NP gene of swine H1N1 influenza virus positive, and the HA gene of type A H1N1 influenza virus positive. By routine blood test, WBC count 3.24×10^9/L, GR% 57.74 %, LY% 32.74 %. Blood biochemistry revealed TP 55 g/L, AST 100U/L, ALT 69U/L, ALB 27 g/L, CK 621U/L, and LDH 511U/L. He experienced persisitent fever during hospitalization with body temperature of 37.4–39.2 °C, cough, expectoration and chest distress. By auscultation, moist rales in both lungs that was more extensive in the right lung. Laboratory test on d 4 after hospitalization, blood routine test revealed WBC count 11.47×10^9/L, GR% 83.01 %, LY% 8.82 %; blood biochemistry revealed TP 55 g/L, A 24 g/L, AST 64U/L, ALT 54U/L, and BUN 3.4 mmol/L.

[Radiological demonstration] Fig. 9.19.

[Diagnosis] Pneumonia induced by type A H1N1 influenza virus.

[Discussion]

Pneumonia is the most common complication of influenza A (H1N1), which is caused by primary viral pneumonia or secondary bacterial infection. Chest HRCT mainly demonstrates diffuse or multiple patches of ground glass opacity in lungs with or with no consolidation, which commonly distribute around bronchovascular tree or in the subpleural area. Pathologically, the lesions are demonstrated as bronchial and peribronchial alveolar congestion, inflammatory exudation, and transparent membrane formation. With the progression of the disease, ground glass opacities rapidly fuse and extend with increased density, with flakes of consolidation in or out of the ground glass opacity; only consolidation but no GGO in some cases.

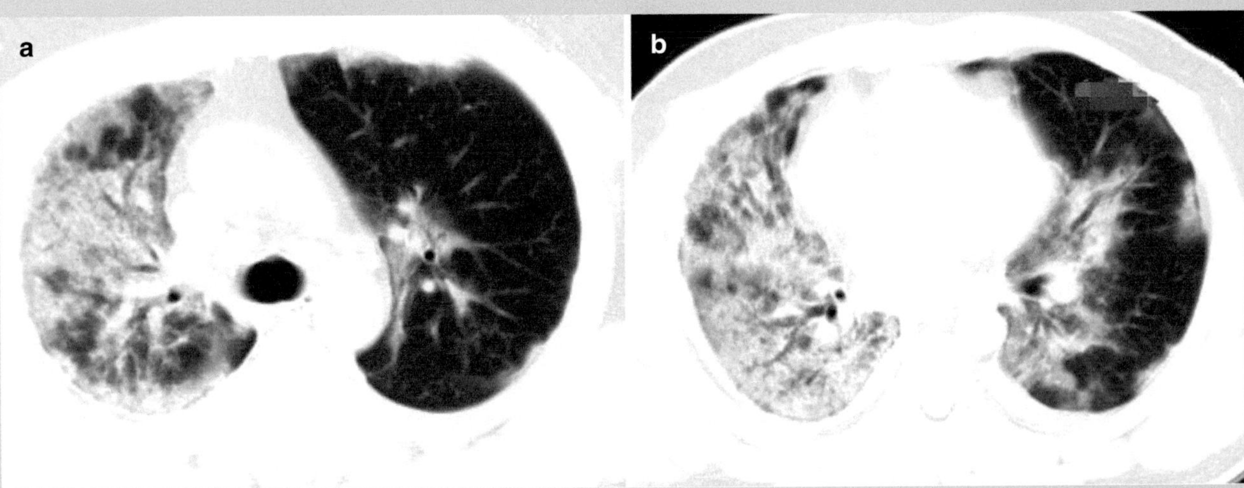

Fig. 9.19 CT scan showed consolidation and ground glass opacity in both lungs, predominantly in the right lung, with air bronchogram inside (**a–d**). Reexaminations after treatment for 4 days showed progression of the lesions in both lungs (**e–h**) (Reprint with permission from Hongjun Li and Ning Li (Eds), Radiology of Influenza A (H1N1), Springer, 2013)

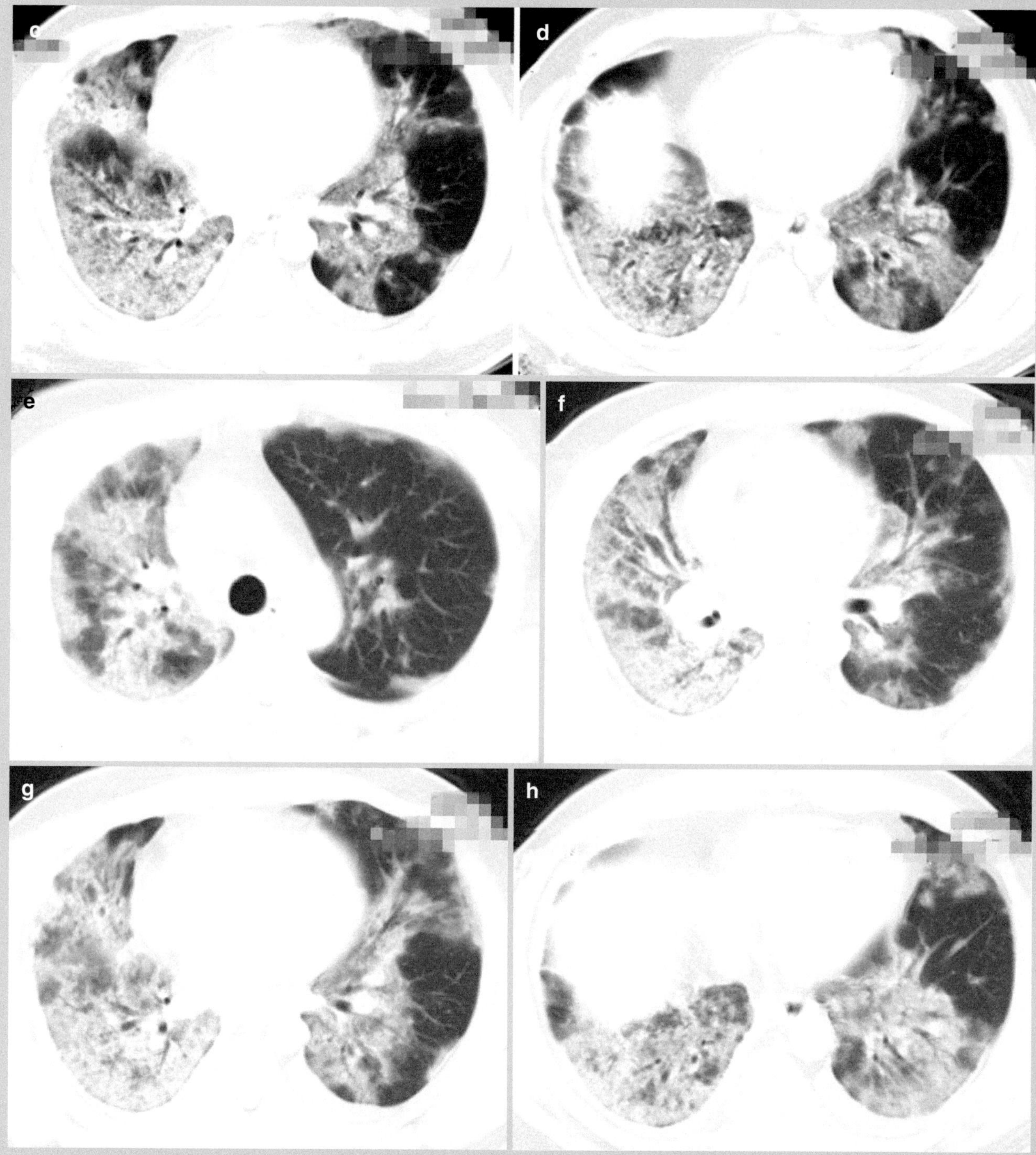

Fig. 9.19 (continued)

Case 20

[Brief Case History]

A 34-year-old woman complained of fever for 7 days and difficulty breathing for 3 days. She experienced cough and expectoration of whitish or yellowish phlegm. The patient denied a history of contact to patient with type A influenza. By physical examination, body temperature 39 °C, pharyngx congested, no tonsilar swelling; coarse breathing sound in both lungs but no moist rales. By laboratory test, the throat swab showed influenza A (H1N1) relalted etiological factors, such as FluA and SWH1, positive.

[Radiological demonstration] Fig. 9.20

[Diagnosis] Pneumonia induced by type A H1N1 influenza virus.

[Discussion]

Radiologically, the lesions in this case were demonstrated as diffuse ground glass opacity, poorly defined hilum in both lungs, and accompanying air trapping. The condition should be differentiated from the following diseases:

1. Mycoplasmal pneumonia
   The lesions are always demonstrated as centri-lobular ground glass density opacity or consolidation, which may develop into lobar or segmental consolidation in a fan like shape. But these lesions are rare in the cases of pneumonia induced by type A H1N1 influenza virus. Mycoplasmal pneumonia in children is radiologically demonstrated as grid like and spots of interstitial lesions, commonly with enlarged hilum and possibly pleural effusion.
2. Chlamydial pneumonia
   The radiological signs of chlamydial pneumonia are non-specific, with flakes of and grid like opacity in unilateral or bilateral lower lung lobes, and the lesions are commonly constrined with slow progression, good mobility and favorable prognosis.

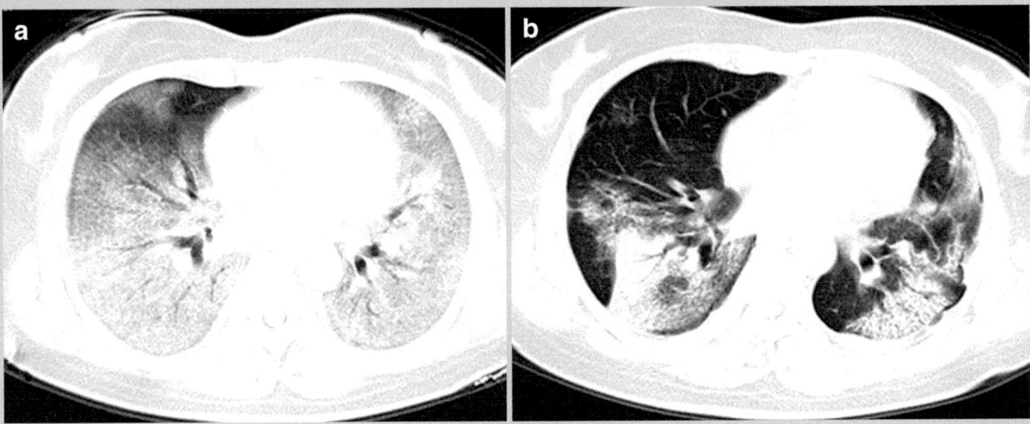

Fig. 9.20 Chest CT scan revealed diffuse ground glass like opacity with high density in both lungs, with air bronchogram inside (**a**). Reexamination after treatment for 18 days revealed cloud and cotton like poorly defined opacity in the left upper lung lobe and bilateral lower lungs lobes; obvious absorption of the lesions (**b**)

Case 21

[Brief Case History]

A 29-year-old man complained of cough for 7 days and fever for 6 days. He also showed wheezing and expectoration of pinkish foamy sputum. By physical examination, the body temperature was 38.6 °C; the pharynx congested; and moist rales in both lungs. He denied a history of contact to patient with type A influenza. By laboratory test, the throat swab showed the M gene of type A influenza virus was positive, the NP gene of swine H1N1 influenza virus positive, and the HA gene of type A H1N1 influenza virus positive. By routine blood test, WBC 2.54×10^9/L, GR% 75.1 %, LY% 15.4 %. Blood gas analysis revealed pH 7.33, PCO_2 54 mmHg, and PO_2 85 mmHg. Blood chemistry revealed ALT

40U/L, AST 32U/L, Cr 115.9 μmol/L, and UREA 16.73 mmol/L. Reexamination after treatment for 9 days, routine blood test showed WBC 7.8×10^9/L, GR% 88.4 %, and LY% 8.2 %; by blood gas analysis, pH 7.512, and PO_2 48.8 mmHg, PCO_2 32.16 mmHg; liver function examination revealed ALT 166.8 IU/L, and AST 270.5 IU/L.

[**Radiological and pathological demonstrations**] Fig. 9.21

[**Diagnosis**] Critical pneumonia induced by type A H1N1 influenza virus.

[**Discussion**]

The patient with critical pneumonia induced by type A H1N1 influenza virus is radiologically demonstrated with multiple large fused consolidations in both lung fields and extensive ground glass opacity around bronchi, which rapidly progressed. The lesions showed great changes even within 1 day and the condition may be complicated by ARDS, pneumothorax, mediastinal and subcutaneous emphysema, even retroperitoneal gas trapping.

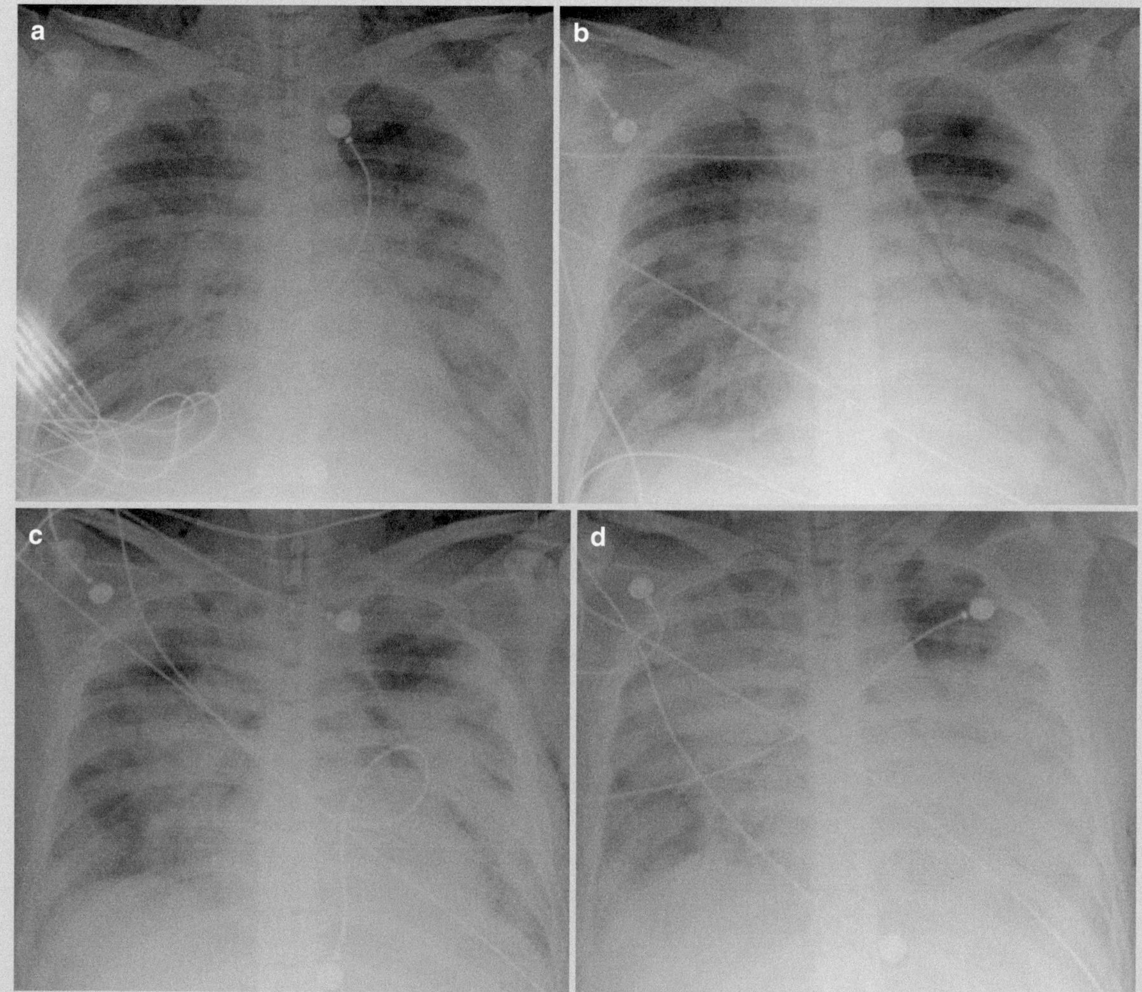

Fig. 9.21 Chest X-ray showed multiple poorly defined flakes of opacity in the bilateral middle and lower lungs fields; enlarged and poorly defined hilum in both lungs; poorly defined bilateral costophrenic angles (**a**). Reexamination after treatment for 1 day revealed progression of the lesions. Chest X-ray showed enlarged range with multiple poorly defined flakes of opacity in the bilateral middle and lower lungs, which showed increased density (**b**). Reexamination after treatments for 4 days, chest X-ray showed enlarged range with consolidations in both lungs (**c**). Reexamination after treatments for 5 days, the lesions were shown with progression (**d**). Reexamination after treatments for 11 days, the lesions were improved and chest X-ray showed poorly defined flakes and cotton like opacity and increased transparency of both lungs (**e**). Pathologically, the alveolus was shown with interlobular septal thickening and alveolar wall congestion; infiltration of neutrophils and plasmocytes, predominantly mononuclear cells; exudation of intra-alveolar edema fluid and fibrin (H&E staining, ×20) (**f**, **g**). Pathologically, the myocardial space was shown with a large quantity of inflammatory cells (H&E staining, ×20) (**h**, **i**) (Reprint with permission from Hongjun Li and Ning Li (Eds), Radiology of Influenza A (H1N1), Springer, 2013)

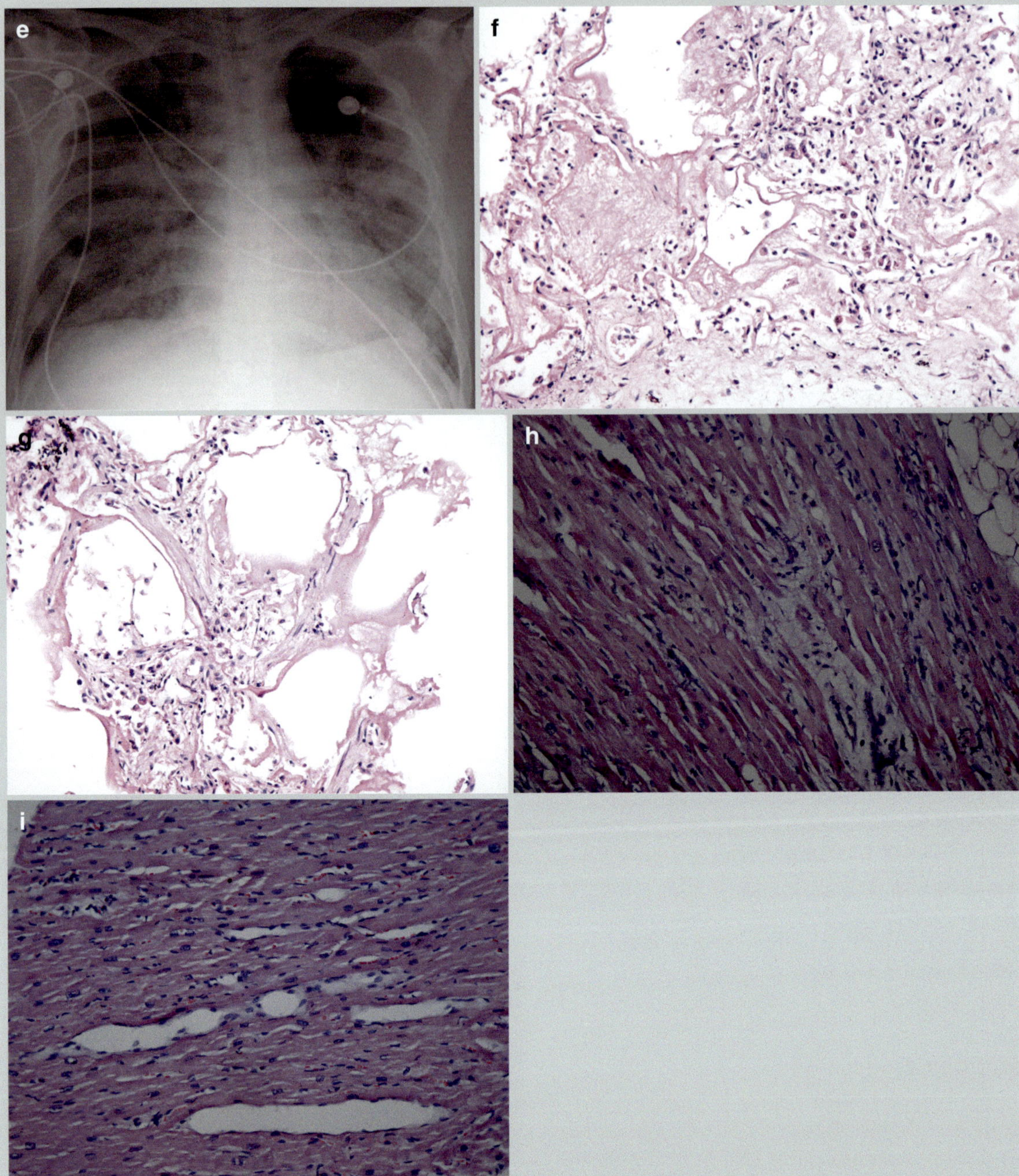

Fig. 9.21 (continued)

Case 22

[**Brief Case History**]

A 21-year-old young woman complained of fever and cough for 9 days. She also experienced cough and expectoration of yellowish sputum, which failed to be improved by anti-inflammatory therapy, with a body temperature fluctuating between 38 °C and 38.7 °C, chest distress, shortness of breath, and expectoration of yellowish sputum. By physical examination, the body temperature 39.7 °C; the pharynx congested; the tonsil swollen in degree I; moist rales in both lungs that were absent after coughs. She reported a non-definitive history of contact to patient with type A influenza. By laboratory test, the throat swab showed that the M gene of type A influenza virus positive, the NP gene of swine H1N1 influenza virus negative, and the HA gene of type A H1N1 influenza virus positive. By routine blood test, WBC 8.64×10^9/L, GR% 76.14%, LY% 19.34%; by blood chemistry, CK 140U/L, and LDH 547U/L.

[**Radiological demonstration**] Fig. 9.22

[**Diagnosis**] Pneumonia induced by type A H1N1 influenza virus and bronchiectasis.

[**Discussion**]

Radiologically, severe pneumonia induced by type A H1N1 influenza virus is demonstrated as the followings: (1) multifocal or diffuse ground glass opacity; (2) multifocal ground glass opacity and consolidation opacity; (3) multifocal or diffuse consolidation; (4) distribution of the lesions in the subpleural lung periphery or around bronchovascular bundles; (5) rapid progression of the lesions into diffuse ground glass opacity or consolidation within 1–3 days.

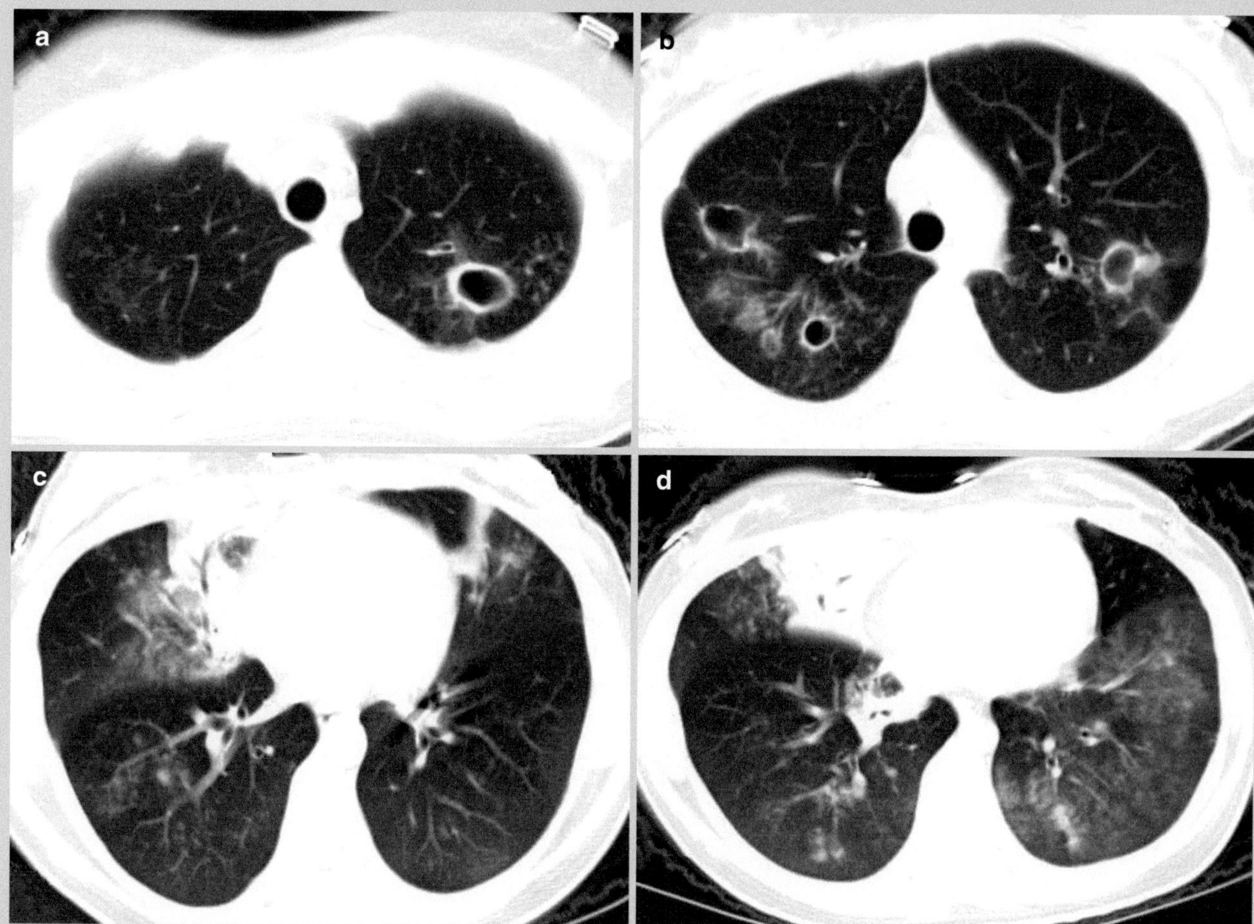

Fig. 9.22 CT scan showed multiple irregular thin-wall cavities in the bilateral upper lung lobes, which was surrounded by sporadic patches of opacity; bronchial wall thickening in the left upper lung lobe, with widened bronchial lumen (**a**, **b**). CT scan showed multiple consolidations and ground glass opacities in both lungs; air bronchogram in consolidation opacity of the medial segment in the right upper lung lobe (**c**, **d**)

Case 23

[Brief Case History]

A 57-year-old woman complained of right upper abdominal pain for 3 days, whose aggravation, chest distress and shortness of breath for 2 days, with disturbance of consciousness. The pain in the right upper quadrant was paroxysmal migratory. She had a medical history of chronic bronchitis for more than 20 years, with long-term use of hormone and edema of lower limbs. She denied medical histories of hypertension and diabetes, but did experienced symptoms of polyphagia, polydipsia and polyuria. The patient reported a history of contact to patient with type A influenza. By physical examination, she was in coma, overweight, ecchymosis all over the body; severe edema of bulbar conjunctiva, conjunctiva hemorrhage in the left eyelid, both pupils in equal size and round being sensitive to light; overwhelming moist rales in both lungs with occasional dry rales; heart rate 102/min, no pathological murmur in each auscultatory valvular regions; abdominal circumference 100 cm, abdominal tension increased; pitting edema inferior to elbow joints of upper limbs and inferior to knees of lower limbs. By laboratory test, the throat swab showed that the M gene of type A influenza virus positive, the NP gene of swine H1N1 influenza virus positive, and the HA gene of type A H1N1 influenza virus positive. By routine blood test, WBC 21.52×10^9/L, GR% 93 %, HGB 139 g/L, PLT 88×10^9/L. Blood gas analysis revealed pH 7.141, PCO_2 19.1 mmHg, PO_2 60 mmHg, SO_2 92 %, BE -22 mmol/L, K^+ 5.2 mmol/L. Blood chemistry revealed ALB 26.7 g/L, GLOB 46 g/L, GLU 42.8 mmol/L, BUN 14.12 mmol/L, osmotic pressure 327 mmol/L. By routine urine test, KET strongly positive (++++), GLU strongly positive (++++). Reexamination after treatment for 1 day, blood gas analysis revealed pH 7.417, PCO_2 48 mmHg, PO_2 100 mmHg, BE 6 mmol/L. Reexamination after treatment for 4 days, by routine blood test, WBC 15.9×10^9/L, GR% 87.5 %, HGB 117 g/L, PLT 113×10^9/L; blood gas analysis revealed pH 7.567, PCO_2 45.5 mmHg, PO_2 74 mmHg, BE 19 mmol/L, HCO^-_3 41.4 mmol/L, SPO_2 96 %; blood chemistry revealed ALT 50U/L, AST 48U/L, ALB 33.2 g/L, GGT 883U/L, PA 136 mg/L, GLU 12.57 mmol/L, GRF 56 ml/min, LACT 2.3 mmol/L. The erythrocyte sedimentation rate 78 mm/h, PT within normal limites, D-dimer positive. Sputum smear revealed negative bacilli in a small quantity, no fungal spore or acid-fast bacillus. By sputum culture, acinetobacter baumannii positive. Reexamination after treatment for 6 days, by routine blood test, WBC 15.5×10^9/L, GR% 88.8 %, PLT 164×10^9/L, HGB 109 g/L; by blood chemistry, ALB 34.4 g/L, PA 158 mg/L, CRP 87.6 mg/L, GLU 10.46 mmol/L, HBDH 255U/L, LDH 357U/L; by blood gas analysis, pH 7.43, PCO_2 64 mmHg, PO_2 67 mmHg, BE 14.9 mmol/L, HCO_3 41.4 mmol/L, FiO_2 60 %, Na^+ 144 mmol/L, and K^+ 3.5 mmol/L. By sputum culture, gram negative bacilli grew in a small quantity. Sputum smear revealed a small amount of positive cocci and negative cocci; a great amount of negative bacilli and fungal spore; D-dimer weakly positive (±). By thoracocentesis, 200 ml dark red bloody pleural fluid was drained.

[Radiological demonstration] Fig. 9.23

[Diagnosis] Pneumonia induced by type A H1N1 influenza virus; right hydropneumothorax; a small quantity of pleural effusion in the left thoracic cavity.

[Discussion]

Severe pneumonia induced by type A H1N1 influenza virus is radiologically characterized by diffuse ground glass opacity and consolidation in the lung periphery of both lungs and their rapid progression. The lesions often progress into diffuse ground glass opacity or consolidation in both lungs within 1–3 days. And the condition is commonly complicated by pneomothorax and mediastinal emphysema. In this case, the lesions in both lungs alternatively aggravated and alleviated, with changes by reexaminations each day. Therefore, the patients with pneumonia induced by type A H1N1 influenza virus should receive chest plain X-ray or CT scan each day during the following-ups for immediate understandings about the progression of the lesions and appropriate treatment.

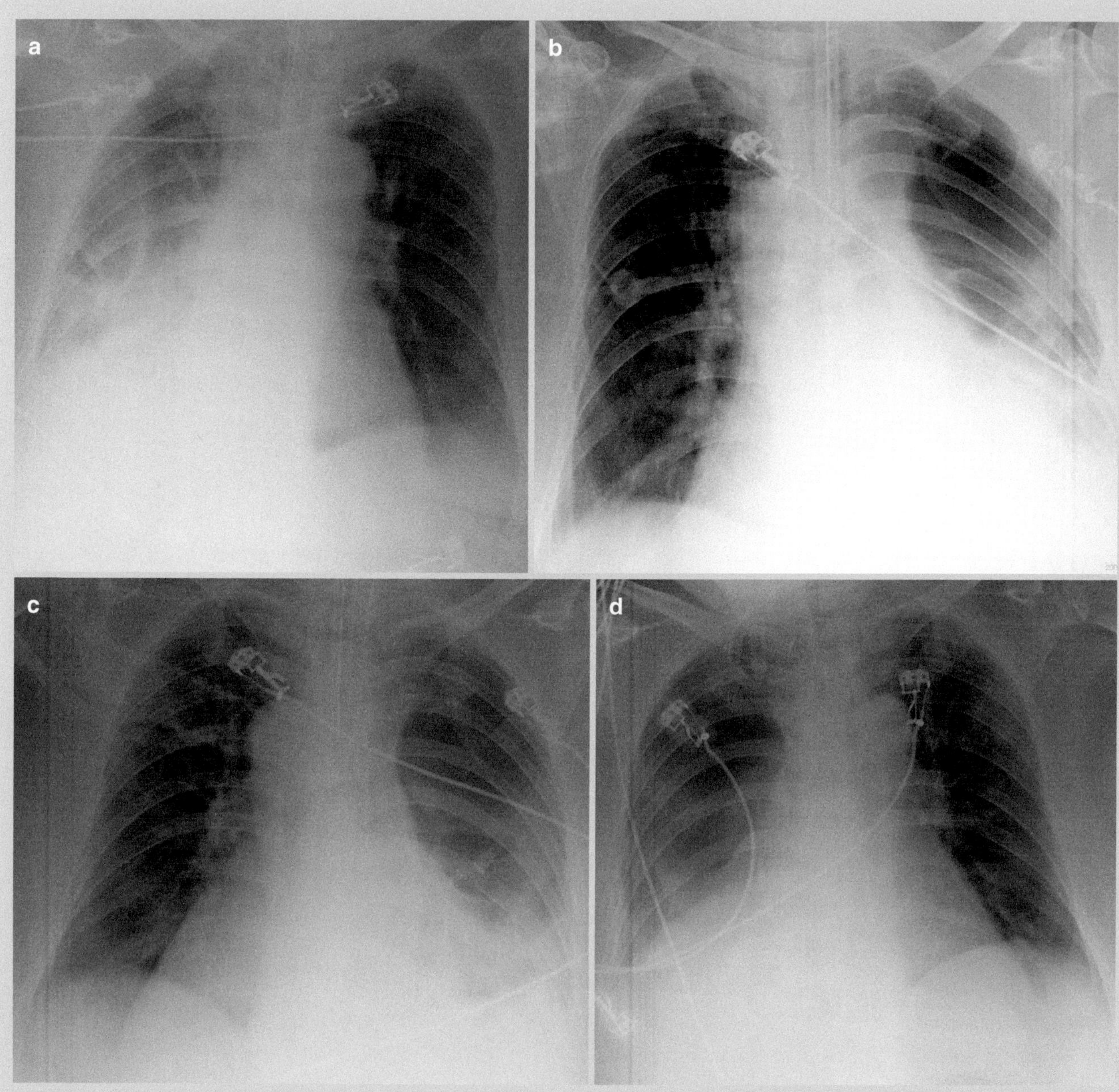

Fig. 9.23 Chest X-ray showed diffuse consolidation in the right middle and lower lung fields and in the left lower lung; poorly defined right diaphragm (**a**). Reexamination after treatment for 2 days, the right lung was shown with increased transparency and sporadic ground glass opacity; the left middle and lower lung fields with consolidation; poorly defined left diaphragm (**b**). Reexamination after treatment for 3 days, the lesions in both lower lungs progressed (**c**). Reexamination after treatment for 4 days, the range with consolidation in the right lung was enlarged; oval shaped area in the right upper lung with no lung markings; smaller range with consolidation in the left lung that showed decreased density (**d**). Reexamination after treatment for 5 days, the range with consolidations in the right lung enlarged; increased density of the consolidation opacity; no change in the area with no lung markings in the right upper lung; multiple light flakes of opacity in the left lung, with thickened lung marking (**e**). Reexamination after treatment for 6 days, the right lung was shown with shrinkage and increased density of the lesions; the left lower lung was shown with multiple cloud like and cotton like consolidation; poorly defined bilateral diaphragm (**f**). Reexamination after treatment for 6 days, CT scan showed consolidation in the right lung and obvious shrinkage of the right lung, with a small amount of normal lung issue; right pneumothorax with air-fluid level; multiple cords like opacity in the left lung and a small quantity of pleural effusion in the left thoracic cavity (**g, h**) (Reprint with permission from Hongjun Li and Ning Li (Eds), Radiology of Influenza A (H1N1), Springer, 2013)

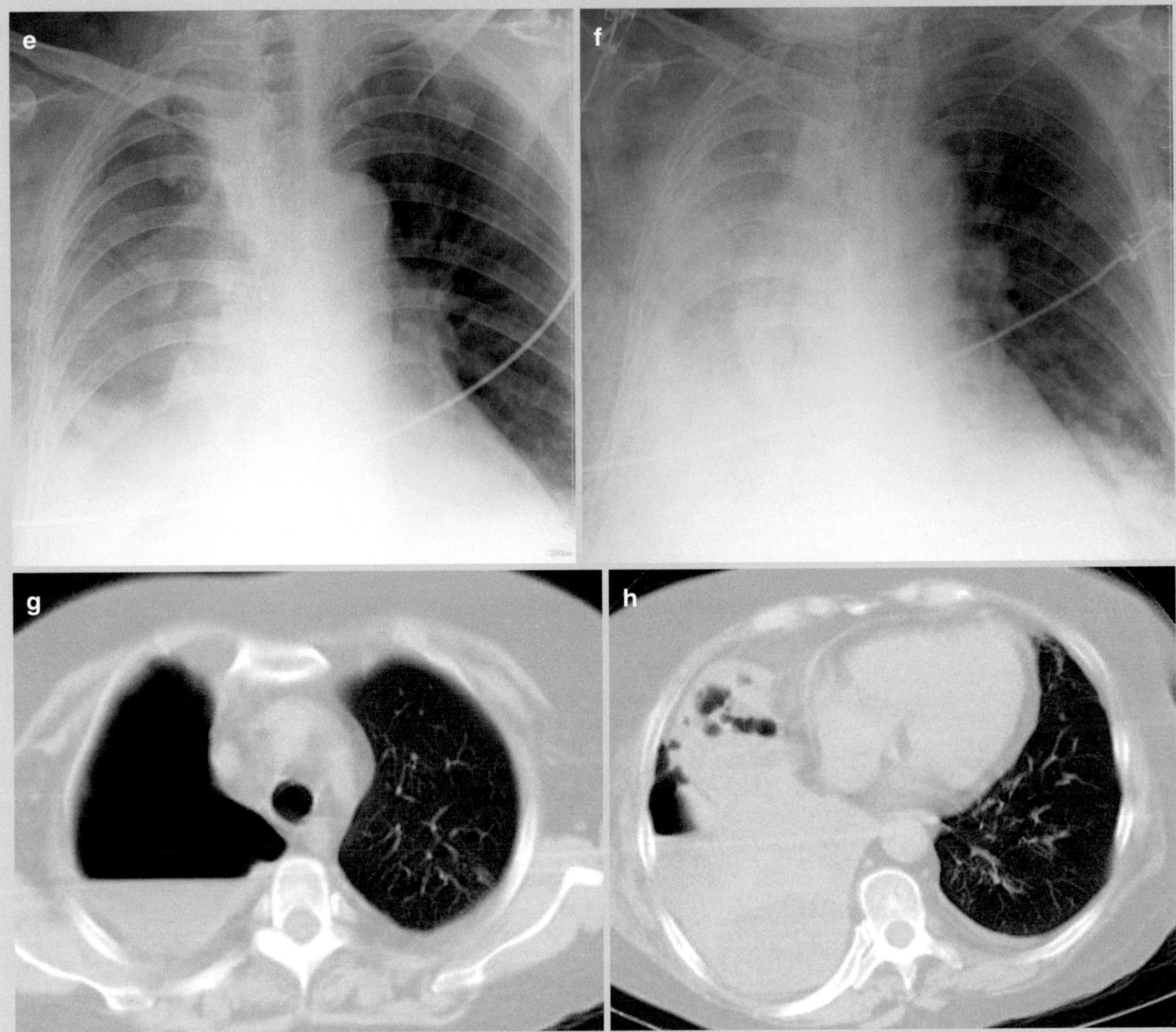

Fig. 9.23 (continued)

Case 24

[Brief Case History]

A 45-year-old woman complained of aversion to cold and fever for 5 days with the highest body temperature of 39.5 °C. She also experienced symptoms of dry cough, expectoration of a small quantity of sputum, chest distress, choking and eye upset. In another hospital, she was diagnosed with bronchitis and was then treated by anti-inflammatory therapy, but showing symptoms of chest distress and shortness of breathing then. After the patient was transferred to our hospital, death occurred due to respiratory failure. She denied a history of contact to patient with type A influenza or patient with flu like symptoms. By physical examination, the body temperature 39 °C and the pharynx congested. By laboratory test, the throat swab showed the M gene of type A influenza virus negative, the NP gene of swine H1N1 influenza virus positive, and the HA gene of type A H1N1 influenza virus positive. By routine blood test, WBC 3.39×10^9/L, GR% 81.1 %, and LY% 14.5 %. Blood gas analysis revealed pH 7.466, PCO_2 35.5 mmHg, and PO_2 76 mmHg. Liver function examination showed ALT 21.1U/L, AST 51.3U/L, UREA 3.34U/L, and CREA 41.0U/L.

[Radiological and pathological demonstrations as well as gross observation] Fig. 9.24

[Diagnosis] Critical pneumonia induced by type A H1N1 influenza virus.

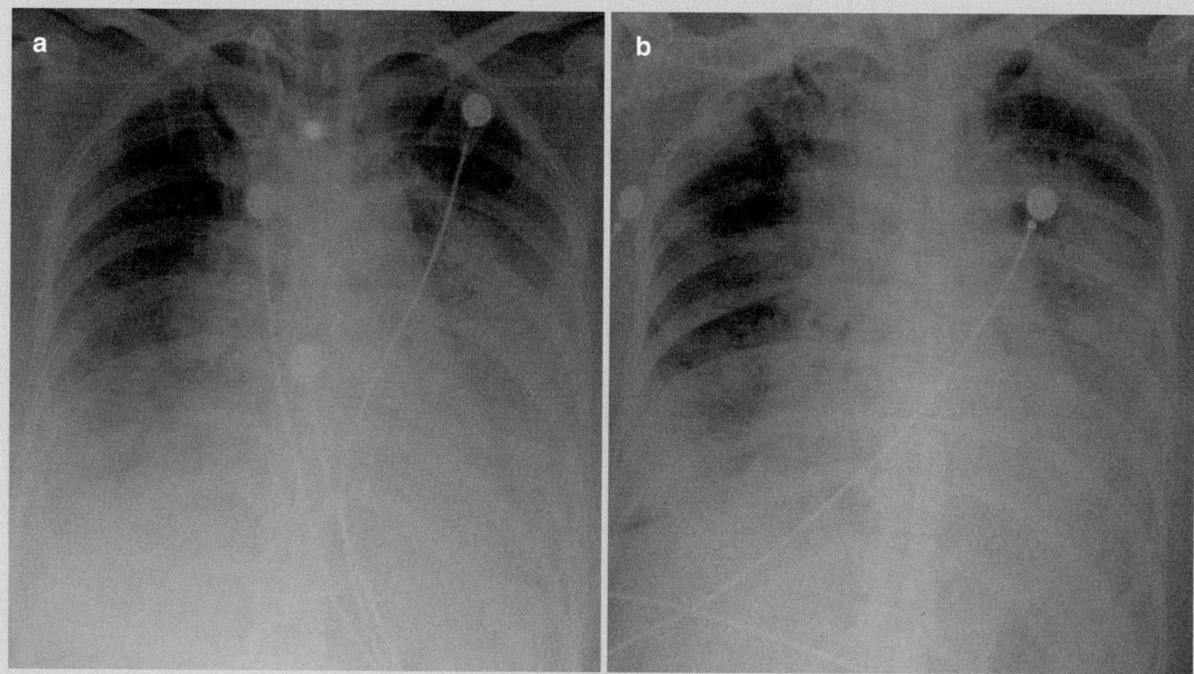

Fig. 9.24 Chest X-ray showed large flakes of poorly defined high density opacity in the middle and lower lung fileds of both lungs; poorly defined bilateral hilum and diaphragm (**a**). Reexamination after treatment for 11 days showed enlarged range with lesions in both lungs and increased density of the lesion (**b**). Reexamination after treatment for 18 days showed diffuse high density opacity in both lungs (**c**). Reexamination after treatment for 32 days showed absorption and improvement of the lesions in both upper lungs (**d**). Reexamination after treatment for 33 days showed increased transparency of the left middle and upper lung fields (**e**). Reexamination after treatment for 34 days showed progression of the lesions in both lungs, in white-lung change (**f**). After treatment for 37 days, death occurred. CT scan after death for 72 h showed rightward shift of the mediastinum, bilateral pleural effusion in large quantities with air-fluid level in the left pleural cavity (**g**). By autopsy after death for 72 h, the gross specimen showed lung tissue fibrosis and patches of hemorrhage (**h**); the microscopic observation showed a small amount of alveolar cells, fibrosis of most lung tissues, many inflammatory cells, and intra-alveolar hemorrhage (H&E staining, ×10) (**i**); a small quantity of alveolar cells, fibrosis of most lung tissues, absence of bronchiolar epithelial cells, a large quantity of inflammatory cells that predominantly macrophages. All of these findings were in consistency with necrotic bronchitis induced diffuse alveolar damages and alveolar hemorrhage (H&E staining, ×40) (**j**); many inflammatory cells in the interhepatocytic space ((**k**) H&E staining, ×10; (**l**) H&E staining, ×40); renal sinus dilation, multiple inflammatory cells in the renal parenchymal space ((**m**) H&E staining, ×10; (**n**) H&E staining, ×40); a small amount of inflammatory cells in the myocardial cells space ((**o**) H&E staining, ×10; (**p**) H&E staining, ×40)

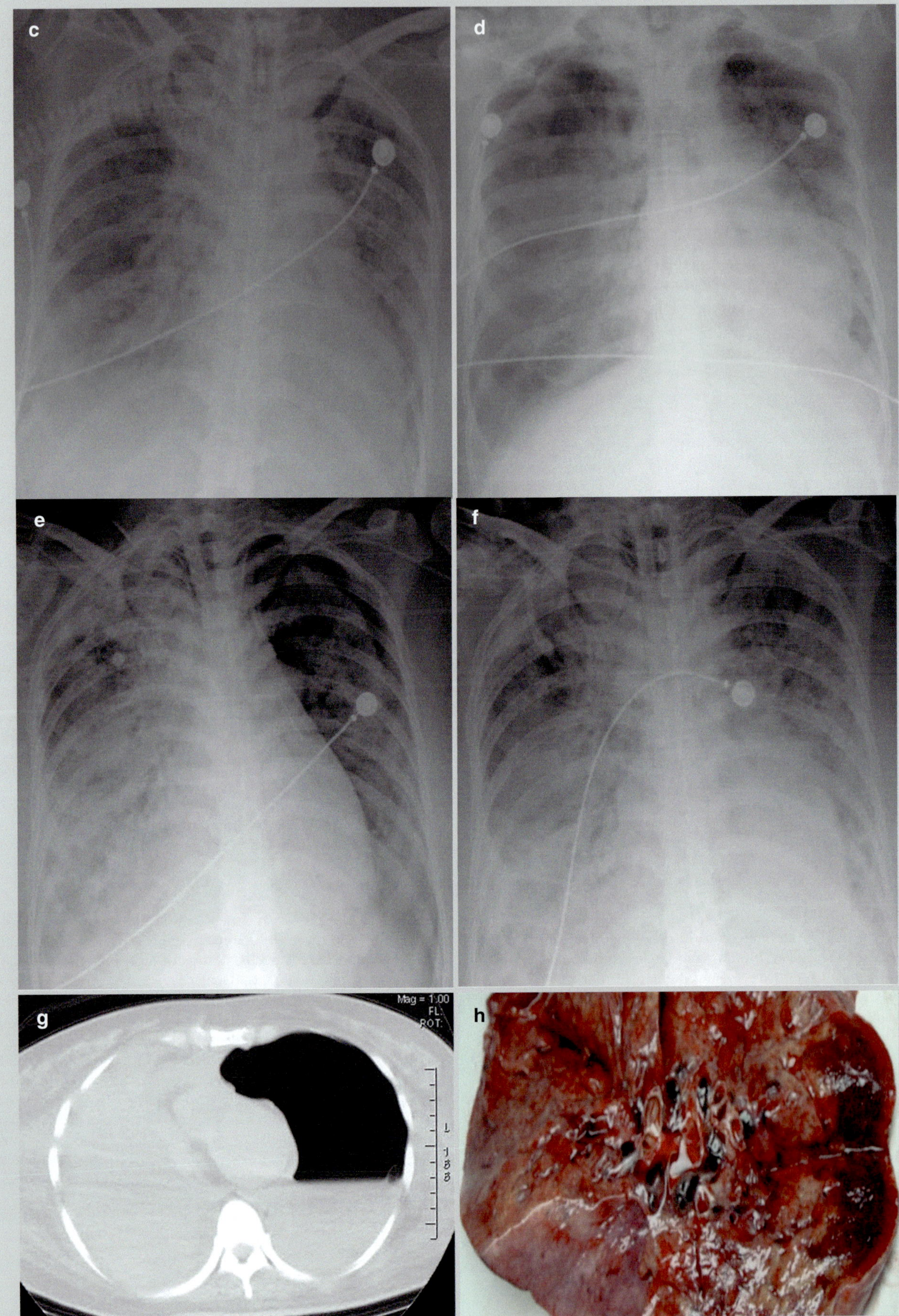

Fig. 9.24 (continued)

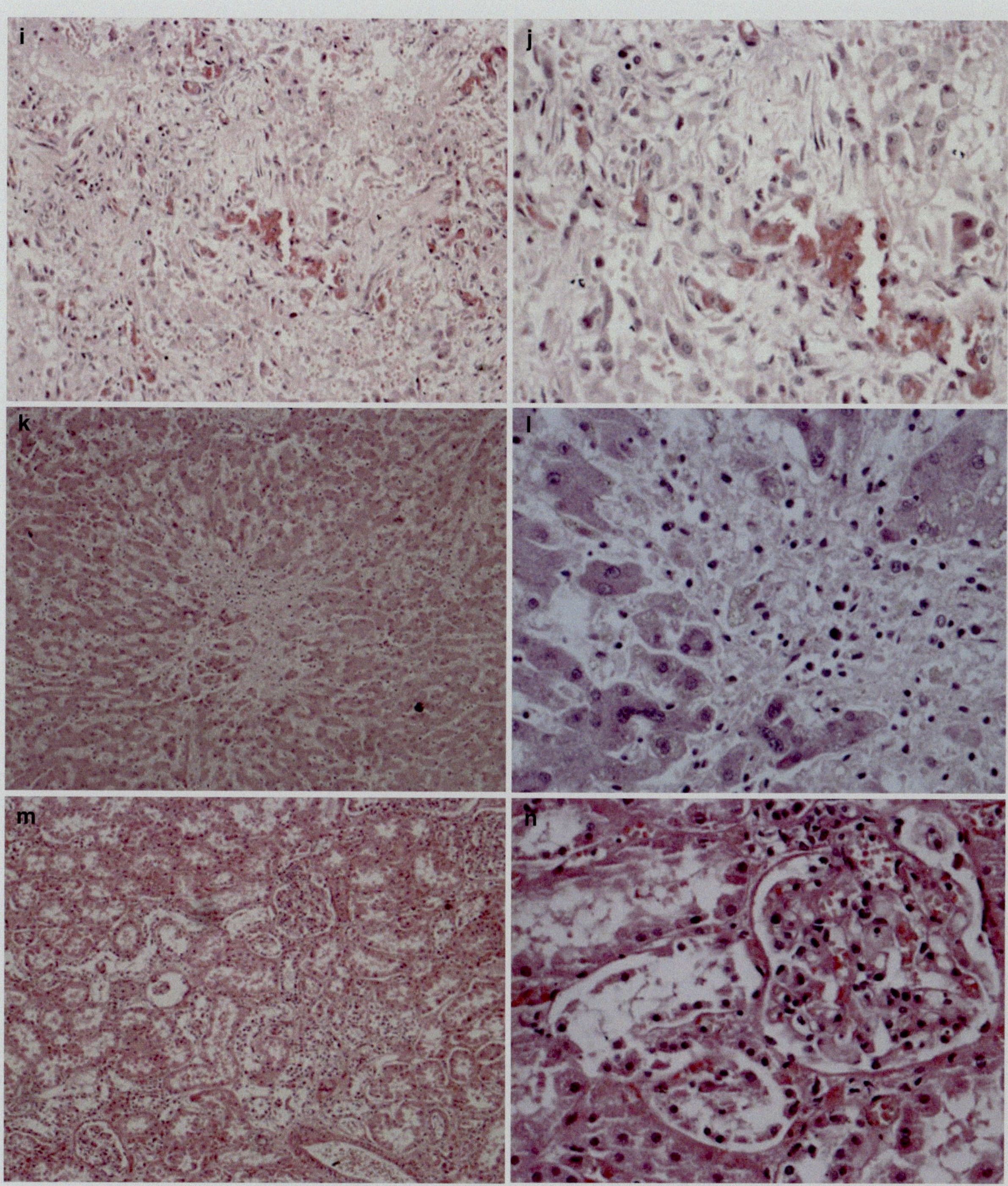

Fig. 9.24 (continued)

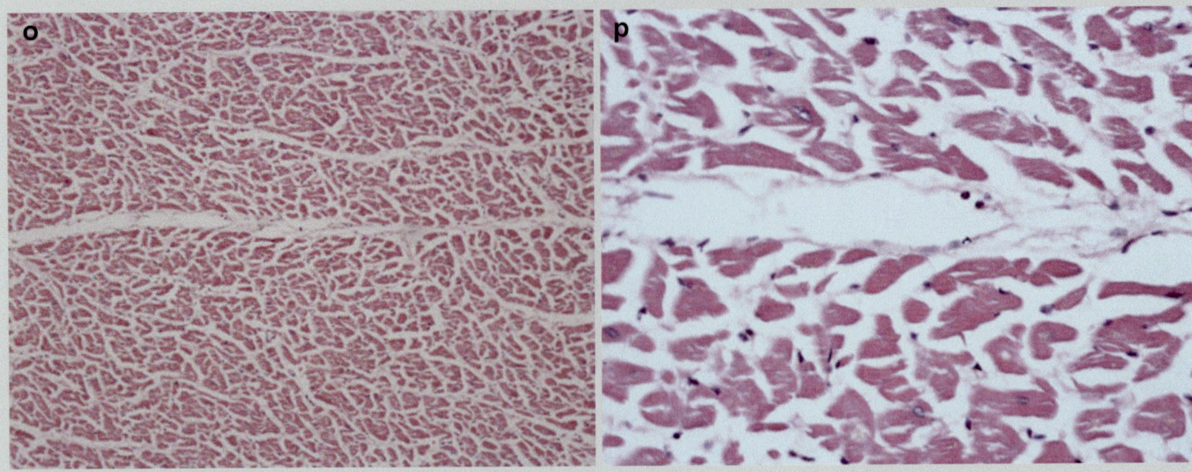

Fig. 9.24 (continued)

Case 25

[**Brief Case History**]

A 48-year-old man complained of fever for 5 days with the highest body temperature of 39 °C. He also experienced expectoration of yellowish thick sputum, shortness of breathing and chest distress. He had medical histories of diabetes, chronic renal insufficiency and chronic bronchitis. He denied a history of contact to patient with type A influenza. By physical examination, the pharynx congested and tonsil swollen in degree I. By laboratory test, the throat swab in laboratory of CDC showed the M gene of type A influenza virus positive, the NP gene of swine H1N1 influenza virus positive, and the HA gene of type A H1N1 influenza virus positive. Routine blood test showed WBC 8.1×10^9/L, RBC 2.49×10^{12}/L. Blood gas analysis revealed pH 7.13, PCO_2 41 mmHg, PaO_2 60 mmHg. Blood chemistry revealed AST 76.3U/L, ALT 13.4U/L. The clinical diagnosis was made as critical influenza A (H1N1). Autopsy was performed after occurrence of death.

[**Pathological demonstration**] Fig. 9.25

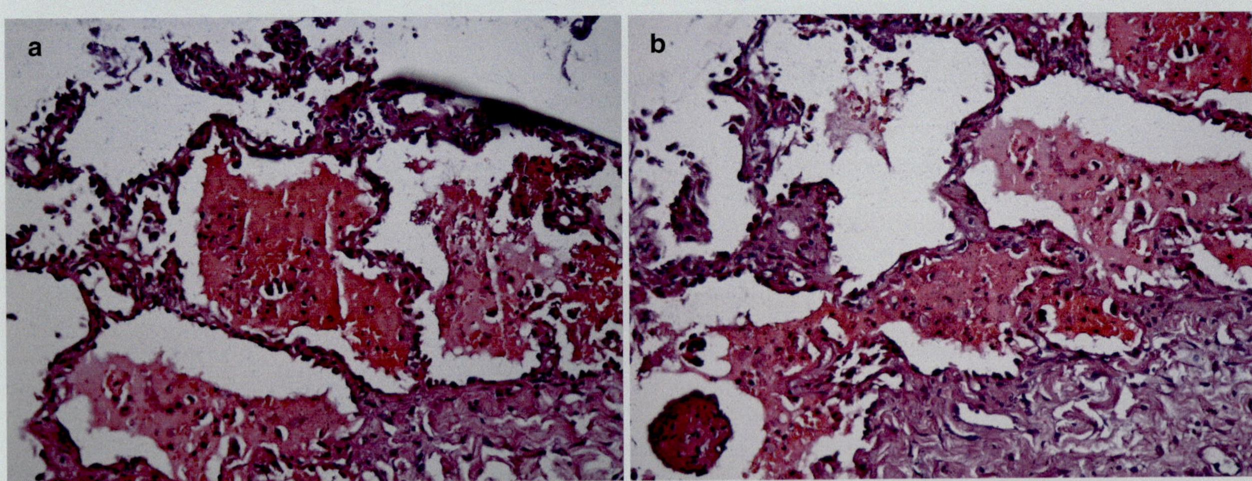

Fig. 9.25 (**a**, **b**) Capillary edema and congestion; infiltration of inflammatory cells ((**a**) H&E staining, ×40; (**b**) H&E staining, ×20); (**c**, **d**) infiltration of a large quantity of inflammatory cells in myocardial tissue ((**c**) H&E staining, ×40; (**d**) H&E staining, ×20)

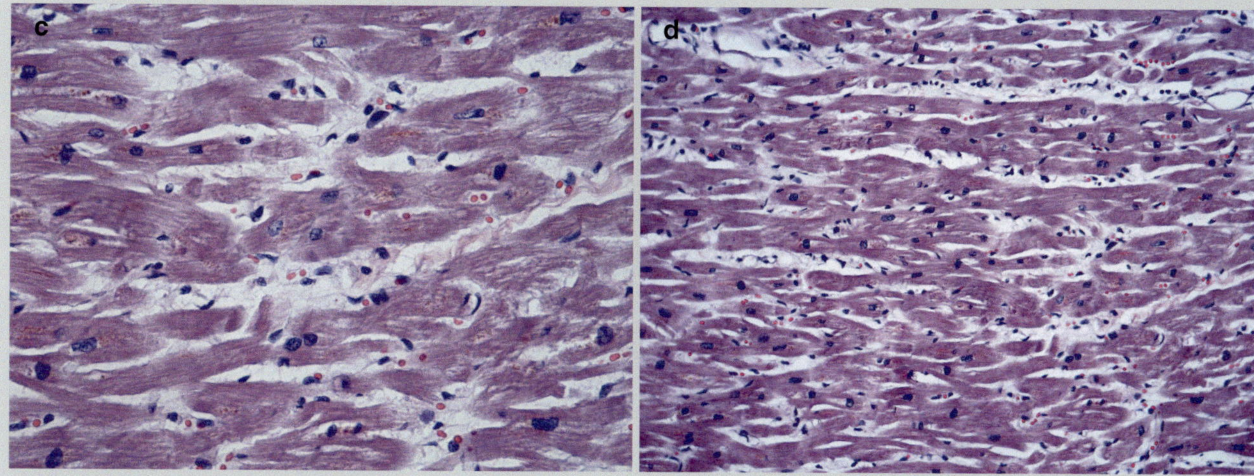

Fig. 9.25 (continued)

References

Abbo L, Quartin A, Morris MI, et al. Pulmonary imaging of pandemic influenza H1N1 infection: relationship between clinical presentation and disease burden on chest radiography and CT. Br J Radiol. 2010;83(992):645–51.

Agarwal PP, Cinti S, Kazerooni EA. Chest radiographic and CT findings in novel swine-origin influenza A(H1N1) virus(S-OIV) infection. AJR. 2009;193(6):1488–93.

Ajlan AM, Quiney B, Nicolaou S, et al. Swine-origin influenza A(H1N1)viral infection: radiographic and CT findings. AJR. 2009;193(6):1494–9.

Americo T, Gino S, Roberto C, et al. Early recognition of the 2009 pandemic influenza A (H1N1) pneumonia by chest ultrasound. Crit Care. 2012;16(1):R30.

Chen F, Zhao DW, Wen S, et al. Radiological demonstrations of severe and critical pneumonia induced by influenza A H1N1 virus. Chin J Radiol. 2010;44(2):123–6.

Cheng H, Duan XM, Peng Y, et al. Chest X-ray and CT scan demonstrations of severe pneumonia induced by influenza A H1N1 virus in children. Chin J Radiol. 2010;44(2):134–6.

Di QG, Li Y, Sun BH, et al. Clinical manifestations of severe influenza A (H1N1) in women during pregnancy. Chin J Tubercu Respir. 2010;33(6):411–4.

Gerardo C, Bertozzi SM, Arantxu CM, et al. Severe respiratory disease concurrent with the circulation of H1N1 influenza. N Engl J Med. 2009;361(7):674–9.

Hu S, Hu CH, Zhang JG, et al. Chest CT scan demonstrations of influenza A (H1N1). J Clin Radiol. 2010;29(6):765–8.

Lee CW, Seo JB, Song JW, et al. Pulmonary complication of novel influenza A(H1N1) infection: imaging features in two patients. Korean J Radiol. 2009;10(6):531–4.

Li HJ. Scientific studies on radiology of influenza A (H1N1) and its related problems. Radiol Pract. 2010;25(9):946.

Li HJ. Radiology of influenza A(H1N1). London: Springer; 2013.

Li HJ, Li N. Radiology of influenza A (H1N1): basic scientific studies and clinical analysis. Beijing: Qinghua University Press; 2011.

Li L, Li HJ. Radiological demonstrations of pneumonia induced by influenza A H1N1 virus. Radiol Pract. 2014;29(7):760–2.

Li HJ, Bao DY, Dai J, et al. Radiological diagnosis and its underlying mechanism of pneumonia induced by influenza A H1N1 virus. Beijing Med. 2010a;32(3):169–72.

Li HJ, Bao DY, Li XQ, et al. Radiological demonstrations and histopathological analysis of critical pneumonia induced by influenza A H1N1 virus. Radiol Pract. 2010b;25(9):951–5.

Li HJ, Li N, Jin RH, et al. Radiological demonstrations and its pathomechanism of lung infection induced by influenza A H1N1 virus. Radiol Pract. 2010c;25(1):100, 101.

Li M, Zhu JB, Chen GQ, et al. Influenza A(H1N1) pneumonia: an analysis of 63 cases by chest CT. Chin Med J (Engl). 2011;124(17):2669–73.

Li HJ, Cheng JL, Li N, et al. Critical influenza (H1N1) pneumonia: imaging manifestations and histopathological findings. Chin Med J (Engl). 2012;125(12):2109–14.

Ma DQ. Value of radiological examinations in the differential diagnosis of lung infections. Chin J Radiol. 2011;45(6):517–9.

Pan JS, Zhang GZ, Cai ZL. Differental diagnosis by chest CT scan. Beijing: Scientific and Technological Literature Press; 2003.

Perez PR. Pneumonia and respiratory failure from swine-origin influenza A(H1N1) in Mexico. N Engl J Med. 2009;361(7):680–9.

Shi YX, Li SJ, Zhou S. Influenza A (H1N1) by chest high-resolution CT scan. Chin J Radiol. 2010;44(2):127–9.

Song CP, Luo H, Bi HJ. Perinatal influenza A (H1N1): report of 12 cases. Forum Primary Med. 2014;18(zl):3–5.

Xie ZP, Dai F, Zhu XQ. Radiological demonstrations of influenza A (H1N1) complicated by ARDS. J Pract Radiol. 2010;26(11):1571–5.

Yang J, Ma DQ. Radiological diagnosis of influenza A (H1N1) complicated by pneumonia. Chin J Radiol. 2010;44(2):219–20.

Zhao GC, Hou KK, Chen Y. Chest CT scan demonstrations of pneumonia induced by influenza A H1N1 virus. Sichuan Med. 2011;32(2):266–7.

Zhong JQ, Chen GP, Peng ZG, et al. Chest X-ray and CT scan demonstrations of influenza A (H1N1). China J Med Radiol Technol. 2011;27(2):317–20.

Zhou M, Guo WL, Wang J. Chest X-ray demonstrations of influenza A (H1N1) in children. Chin J Radiol. 2011;45(6):530–2.

Zhou L, Liu Q, He YL, et al. CT scan demonstrations of influenza A (H1N1). J Nanchang Univ (Edition of Medicine). 2012;52(2):52–4.

Zhu YC, Wang JL, Liu LH, et al. Chest CT scan demonstrations of severe influenza A (H1N1): report of 6 cases. China J Med Radiol. 2011;19(2):149–52.

10 Human Infected H5N1 Avian Influenza

Puxuan Lu, Boping Zhou, Jing Yuan, and Guilin Yang

10.1 Introduction

10.1.1 Definition and Prevalence

Avian influenza is an infectious disease caused by avian influenza virus, which is also known as avian plague or European avian plague.

The influenza virus that infects poultry is known as avian influenza virus (AIV), which is categorized into the genus of influenza virus A and the family of Orthomyxoviridae. Currently, AVI is categorized into 16 H subtypes (H1 ~ H16) and 9 N subtypes (N1 ~ N9) according to the respective antigenicity of hemagglutinin (HA) and neuramidinase (NA). In addition to poultry, AVI can also infect I human, pig, horse, mink and marine mammals. According to the varying virulence of AVI to chicken, it is graded into highly pathogenic, moderately pathogenic and mildly or non-pathogenic.

Human infected H5N1 avian influenza is an acute respiratory infectious disease caused by avian influenza virus (H5N1). It is also known as highly pathogenic avian influenza (HPAI) due to its serious symptoms and high mortality. The 1 case of human infected H5N1 avian influenza, a 3-year-old child, was reported in Hong Kong on May 5, 1997. The child was hospitalized due to cold and fever but incurable by therapies, and death occurred due to Reye syndrome and multiple organs failure 10 days after the onset. On May 9, 1997, a strain of H5N1 AIV, nominated as A/Hongkong/157/97, was isolated from his tracheal secretion in National Central Laboratory of Influenza in Rotterdam, Holland and Center for Disease Control, the United States. Therefore, the child was etiologically diagnosed with human infected H5N1 avian influenza. And the child was the first case of human infected highly pathogenic avian influenza (H5N1). Within the following 6 months, 17 other cases were reported, and the patients aged 1–60 years, with the same H5N1 virus strain isolated from their respiratory secretions. In December, 1997, AIV H5N1 was isolated in samples collected from a market selling alive poultry. By killing sick poultry in a large-scale, human infection was then rapidly controlled. In the year of 1997, a total of 18 cases human infected H5N1 avian influenza were reported, with 5 cases of death.

Since the first occurrence of human infected H5N1 avian influenza in HongKong in 1997, a total of 667 cases have been definitively diagnosed globally, with 393 cases of death by Dec. 31, 2014. And the death rate was 58.92 %. WHO warned that human infected H5N1 avian influenza may be one of the most potentially life-threatening diseases and should be highly concerned across the world.

10.1.2 Epidemiology

10.1.2.1 Source of Infection

The infected poultry by AIV H5N1 or the poultry carrying AIV H5N1, such as chicken, duck, goose, and dove, particularly chicken, are important sources of its infection. Wild aquatic birds (mostly with in apparent infection) play an important role in natural spread of the disease. Birds, such as swallow, chukar, bar-headed goose, crow, sparrow, and heron, may also act as the source of its infection. And migration of migrant birds also contributes to the transmission of AIV. Evidence is still needed to prove whether human is also a source of its infection.

10.1.2.2 Route of Transmission

Respiratory Transmission

Route of respiratory transmission refers to inhalation of droplets and droplet nuclei carrying pathogenic AIV particles. AIV infection spreads via airborne transmission, and human can be infected after direct contact to sick poultry or asymptomatic infected poultry, their secretions

P. Lu (✉) • B. Zhou • J. Yuan • G. Yang
Affiliated Shenzhen Third People's Hospital, Guangdong Medical College, Shenzhen, Guangdong, China
e-mail: lupuxuan@126.com

H. Li (ed.), *Radiology of Influenza*, DOI 10.1007/978-94-024-0908-6_10

and excretions. Otherwise, human can also be infected after exposure to the contaminated environment by AIV. After such direct contact or exposure, the virus particles are inhaled into and attached to human upper respiratory tract for further invasion.

Contact Transmission

Transmission via direct or indirect contact refers to human infection of H5N1 avian influenza after close contact to feces of poultry/animal infected by AIV H5N1. Via direct or indirect contact, the virus can be inoculated into human upper respiratory tract, conjunctival mucosa or skin wound by itself.

Susceptible Population

The data from the cases with human infected H5N1 avian influenza indicated that human infected H5N1 avian influenza affects any age group and children under the age of 12 years shows a higher incidence with no gender difference. In addition, the patients from such an age group commonly experience serious conditions.

In addition, human infected H5N1 avian influenza can also spread via other routes of transmission, including gastrointestinal tract, skin wound, conjunctiva, aerosol, and blood. It may also spread vertically or in laboratory, traffic vehicle, and hospital.

10.1.3 Clinical Manifestation

In the early stage of human infected H5N1 avian influenza, the patients commonly experience common influenza like symptoms, including fever with a body temperature persistently above 39 °C with accompanying runny nose, nasal obstruction, cough, sore throat, headache, muscular soreness and general malaise. And some patients may experience gastrointestinal symptoms including nausea, abdominal pain, and diarrhea of watery loose stools. In serious cases, the patients show persistent high fever that rapidly progresses into obvious pneumonia, acute lung injury (ALI), acute respiratory distress syndrome (ARDS), pulmonary hemorrhage, pleural effusion, multiple organ failure, disseminated intravascular coagulation (DIC), shock, and Reye syndrome. Secondary bacterial infection may also occur to complicate the disease that progresses into septicemia, with a mortality of up to above 50 %.

10.1.4 Radiological Demonstration

Due to virus infiltration, the lung of patients with human infected H5N1 avian influenza is demonstrated with flakes of opacity that is predominantly exudates by chest X-ray or chest CT scan, namely the ground glass opacity and lung consolidation. In serious cases, the lesions in lungs progress rapidly, radiologically demonstrated as large ground glass opacity and lung consolidation. In the advanced stage, both lungs are shown with diffuse consolidation.

Human infected H5N1 avian influenza is radiologically characterized by:

1. Early increased density opacity and ground glass opacity in upper lung field

   In the early stage after onset, the upper lung field is demonstrated with flakes of increased density opacity and ground glass opacity, which are the radiological signs of human infected avian influenza.
2. Diffuse lesion

   The invasion of H5N1 avian influenza virus to human lung tissues causes an extensive range of lesions, with diffuse and exudative lesions in multiple lobes and multiple segments of both lungs. At the peak of their progression, most of lung fields in both lungs are involved, with large flakes of cloudy dense mass like opacity or even white-lung sign.
3. Rapid changes of the lesion

   Radiologically, the lesions are demonstrated with rapid changes. A lesion that is initially found in one lung field may rapidly develop to involve the upper, middle and lower lung fields within 24–48 h, radiologically demonstrated as involvement of the whole lung lobe.
4. Concurrently involved pulmonary parenchyma and interstitium

   Due to necrosis and shedding of pulmonary alveoli, the pulmonary alveoli contain less gas but are filled with exudates such as various serous fluids, fibrin, erythrocytes, and neutrophilic granulocytes. In addition, hyaline membrane obviously forms in the alveolar space. Therefore, the lesions of human infected H5N1 avian influenza are radiologically demonstrated as alveolar exudates and lung consolidation, with the involved exudative lesions overlapping with pulmonary interstitium. After the exudative lesions are absorbed, grid like, flakes, strips and patches of opacity is shown, which resemble to the radiological signs of viral pneumonia.
5. Slow absorption of the lesion

   The lesions are slowly absorbed. After the invasive assisting mechanical ventilation is retrieved with subsequent normal body temperature, breathing rate and WBC count, the both lungs are still radiologically demonstrated with strips, flakes, grid like, and patches of consolidation opacity, indicating inconsistency between chest radiology and clinical symptoms due to long-term progression of the lesions. That is to say, the absorption of lesions in lung lags behind clinical manifestations. In adult patients, the pleura is involved in different degrees, with a small quantity of pleural effusion isolateral to the primary lesion as well as bilateral pleural thickening and adhesion. During the absorption stage, multiple lesions of lobular paraseptal emphysema are revealed, with no obvious signs of hilar and mediastinal lymphadenectasis.

10.2 Typical Cases

Case 1

[Brief Medical History]

A 31-year-old male truck driver experienced fever, cough and shortness of breath since Jun. 3, 2006. After he paid a clinic visit in a local hospital, a diagnosis was made to be common cold and he received corresponding therapy. At 0:30 a.m. on Jun. 10, 2006, he was hospitalized due to aggravated condition. By physical examination, the body temperature was 39.2–40 °C, heart rate 127/min, breathing rate 32/min and blood pressure 116/80 mmHg. He showed a typical development, moderate nutrition, active position and slight unconsciousness. In addition, he showed eye conjunctival congestion and edema, identically sized and round pupils and obvious cyanosis in oral lips. By percussion, the left lung flatness; by auscultation, coarse breathing sound of both lungs that attenuated at the right lung. At d 15 prior to the onset, his wife ever went to buy an alive chicken at a market and brought it back home after having it killed on site. His wife and daughter showed no signs of pneumonia. By routine blood test, WBC 4.20×10^9/L, N 0.75, L 0.24, HGB 127 g/L, RBC 4.84×10^{12}/L, PLT 132×10^9/L. By blood glass analysis, pH 7.426, PaO_2 63 mmHg, $PaCO_2$ 34 mmHg, SO_2% 92 %. By blood biochemistry, GLU 7.87 mmol/L, BUN 2.8 mmol/L, Cr 88 μmol/L, ALT 30U/L, and AST 66U/L. T cell count in peripheral blood was 5/μl. Etiologically, RT-PCR by QIAGEN One Step RT-PCR kit was performed to examine his tracheal secretions. The examination report indicated that the target segments of H5 and N1 were amplified. Throat swab for RNA of H5N1 (PCR) twice were positive. All the above findings indicated the existence of H5N1 avian influenza virus.

[Radiological demonstration] See Fig. 10.1

[Diagnosis] Human infected H5N1 avian influenza complicated by pneumonia.

[Discussion]

Following the first case of human infected H5N1 avian influenza reported in HongKong in 1997, 6 cases of death were subsequently reported. By Dec. 31, 2014, a total of 40 cases was reported in China, with 27 cases of death, and the mortality was up to 67 %. The high death rate indicated strong virulence of avian influenza virus H5N1 and the rapid progression of the disease. Chest radiological examinations are of great importance for our understandings about its radiological demonstrations, which facilitate its diagnosis, differential diagnosis and treatment.

Via systematic examination as well as dynamic observation and analysis, the radiological demonstrations and all the dynamic changes of the lesions were harvest from the patient. The radiological demonstrations are characterized by:

1. On d 7 after onset, the first chest X-ray demonstrated large flakes of increased density opacity in the left upper and middle lung fields. On d 8 after onset, the first chest CT scan demonstrated large consolidation opacity with high density in the apico-posterior and anterior segments of the left lung and in the left lower lung lobe, with air bronchogram inside. The anterior segment of the right upper lung was shown with ground glass opacity. All the findings indicated that ground glass opacity and large consolidation opacity are early signs of human infected avian influenza by chest radiology.
2. The invasion of human lung tissues by avian influenza virus H5N1 is extensive, demonstrated as diffuse and exudates lesions in both lungs with multiple segments and lobes involved. At the peak of its progression, most of the lung fields in both lungs is involved, demonstrated as large cloudy dense mass like opacity and even white-lung sign.
3. Radiologically, the lesions change rapidly. The initial lesions in the left upper and middle lung fields can extend into the left lower lung field within 24 h to involve the whole lung. In the following 48 h, the lesions may rapidly extend into the right upper, middle and lower lung fields to involve the whole lungs.
4. The lesions are absorbed slowly. In this case, on d 35 after onset, the invasive assisting mechanical ventilation was retrieved, and the patient subsequently showed normal body temperature, breathing rate and WBC count. On d 33 after onset, chest CT scan still showed strips, flakes, grid like and patches of consolidation opacity with obvious air bronchogram inside. The follow-up CT scan was then performed each year, and the 5th chest CT scan showed interstitial fibrosis in both lungs, demonstrated as lobular septal thickening, sub-pleural arc shape linear opacity, paraseptal emphysema, ground glass opacity, bronchoectasis and small consolidation opacity.
5. The pleura is involved in different degrees. Pleural effusion in a small quantity was demonstrated isolateral to the primary lesions, and bilateral pleura were shown to be thickened with adhesion.

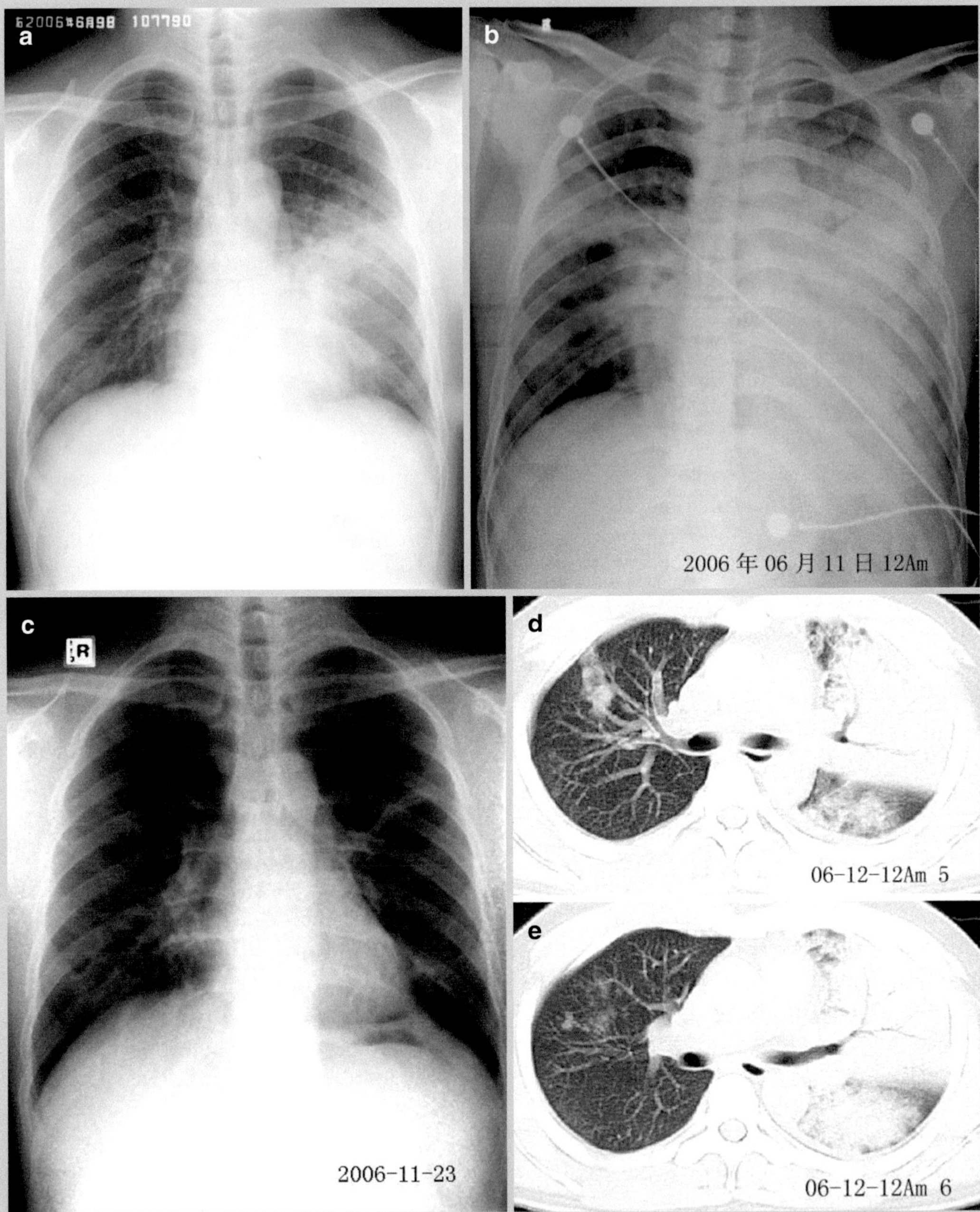

Fig. 10.1 (**a**) On d 6 after onset, chest X-ray demonstrated poorly defined large flakes of increased density opacity at the left middle and lower lung fields, and some of the lesions showed ground glass opacity. (**b**) On d 8 after onset, chest X-ray reexamination demonstrated rapid progression of the lesions, with large flakes of increased density opacity at the whole left lung fields in white-lung sign. Flakes of increased density opacity were revealed at the right hilum area of right middle lung field and middle-medial zone of right lower lung field. (**c**) On d 20 after onset, chest X-ray reexamination demonstrated sporadic spots and cords like increased density opacity in both lungs, with well defined boundaries. (**d, e**) On d 7 after onset, CT scan showed light small flakes of opacity at the posterior segment of right upper lung lobe and medial segment of the right middle lung lobe. Irregular small flakes of consolidation was revealed at the apico-posterior segment and anterior segment of left upper lung lobe. Large flake of dense opacity of consolidation was also revealed at the lingual segment of the upper lung lobes and most of the lower lung lobes, with air brochogram inside. Left pleural effusion was also demonstrated in a moderate quantity. (**f, g**) On d 34 after onset, CT scan showed ground glass opacity at the apical and posterior segments of right upper lung lobe, patches of consolidation at the anterior segment of right upper lung lobe with air bronchogram inside, comparatively shrinkage of the right middle lung lobe in dense opacity of consolidation with air bronchogram inside. The right lower lobe was revealed with scattering irregular patches of opacity, fine arch like linear opacity dorsally near the pleura, and slight thickening of the adjacent pleura. The left upper lung lobe was demonstrated with generally increased density opacity with air bronchogram inside and surrounding lobular septal thickening that reaches subpleura. The lower lung lobe showed slightly small volume, with aggregating lung markings, extensive consolidation and thick air bronchogram inside. (**h, i**) On d 286 after onset, CT scan revealed the lesions in lungs to be pulmonary interstitial changes including fibrous cords like, grid like and ground glass opacity

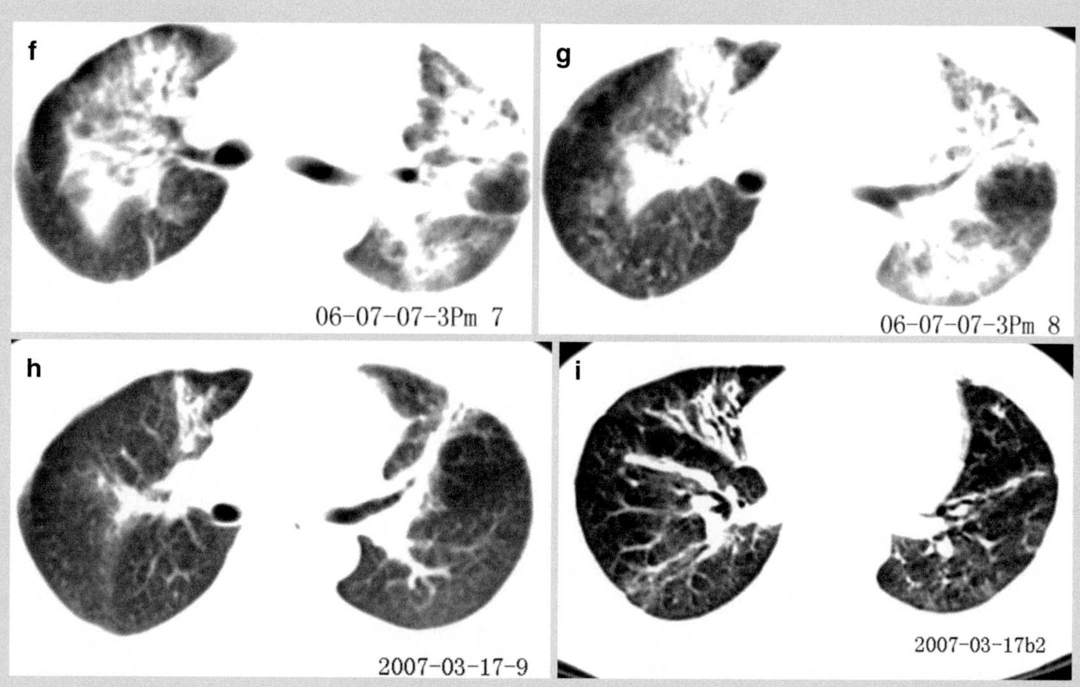

Fig. 10.1 (continued)

The occurrence complications following human infected avian influenza is the direct cause of death and should be highly concerned in clinical practice. The common complications and their prognoses are described as the following:

1. Acute respiratory distress syndrome (ARDS)

   In the most serious stage of the disease, extensive consolidation opacity in both lungs, namely the white–lung sign, indicates the occurrence of ARDS. In this cases, the patient showed the sign of ARDS on d 9 after onset. After invasive mechanical positive pressure ventilation and anti-anoxia therapy were administered, his condition was improved. And multiple organs dysfunction syndrome (MODS) was controlled.
2. Pulmonary secondary infection

   Common pulmonary secondary infections include pseudomonas aeruginosa infection, mycotic infection and other bacterial infections. Since d 10 after onset, the patient was detected for several times with growth of pseudomonas aeruginosa in his phlegm specimens. Particularly on d 20 after onset, his WBC count obviously increased and chest X-ray demonstrated patches uneven opacity in the left lower lung. After polymyxin B and other medications were administered, his pulmonary secondary infection was controlled.
3. Pulmonary fibrosis

   Although his condition was stable with normal vital signs, on discharge his both lungs were shown with irregular grid like, fibrous strips and patches of opacity and accompanying local pleural thickening by thin layer CT scan. These findings indicated existence of pulmonary fibrosis, whose underlying mechanism may be hyperplasia of fibrous tissues and capillaries caused by fibrosis and organization of exudates as well as formation of microthrombosis in pulmonary capillaries based on formation of alveolar hyaline membrane and fibrin exudation. However, the hypothesis needs to be proved by sufficient evidence and the dynamic changes of pulmonary fibrosis still need to be further studied.
4. Pleural effusion

   In this case, the patient showed left pleural effusion in a small quantity on d 8 after onset by the first chest CT scan. On d 33 after onset, the second chest CT scan demonstrated absorption of pleural effusion as well as local pleural thickening and adhesion. These findings indicated pleura is involved in patients with human infected avian influenza, which has been further proved by autopsy.

H5N1 avian influenza should be differentiated from the following diseases.

1. Severe acute respiratory syndrome (SARS)

The lung changes of both human infected avian influenza and SARS are mainly parenchymal and interstitial lesions, with similar shape, development and outcome. Therefore, their differential diagnosis is challenging, and depends mainly on etiological examination and epidemiological history.

SARS is an acute respiratory infectious disease caused by novel corona virus. At its early stage, radiology demonstrates pulmonary interstitial changes, predominantly ground glass opacity. During its progressive stage, the lesions are demonstrated as predominantly ground glass opacity and rarely large consolidation opacity. The lung lesions of human infected H5N1 avian influenza show rapid changes. In some serious patients, the lesions in lungs may change within several days or even 1 day, with rapid progression from small area to large area, from upper or lower lung to the whole lung, from one lung to both lungs, and from ground glass opacity to consolidation opacity. However, in patients with SARS, the lesions in lungs progress slowly, and some lesions are migratory.

The lesions of human infected H5N1 avian influenza are in one lung or both lungs, possibly in upper and lower lung. In serious cases, the lesions are diffuse in both lungs, with more serious condition at the lower lungs. However, in the early stage of SARS, the nodular lesions are commonly located in the subpleural lateral lung field.

2. Type A viral pneumonia

Based only on radiological findings, pneumonia induced by H5N1, H1N1 and H7N9 avian influenza viruses can hardly be differentiated. And their differential diagnosis is mainly based on epidemiological history and etiological examination.

Pneumonia induced by H1N1, H5N1 and H7N9 avian influenza virus is caused by influenza A virus, with clinical influenza like manifestations. Chest CT scan demonstrates the diseases with ground glass opacity and consolidation opacity of varying sizes. Compared to pneumonia induced by H1N1 avian influenza virus, the lesions of pneumonia induced by H5N1 and H7N9 avian influenza virus are radiologically demonstrated with a larger range, with more rapid progression and more common air bronchogram. The lesions of pneumonia induced by H5N1 avian influenza virus show the more rapid progression, followed by H7N9 and then H1N1.

By chest CT scan, pneumonia induced by H5N1 avian influenza virus is demonstrated with large ground glass opacity and consolidation opacity in both lungs that distribute extensively and progress rapidly. In some cases, the lesions are migratory, with slow absorption and obvious pulmonary interstitial fibrosis. Its mortality rate is around 60 %. Pneumonia induced by H7N9 avian influenza virus is radiologically demonstrated with initial lesions in bilateral middle and lower lungs that are predominantly ground glass opacity and consolidation opacity. These lesions show rapid progression and relatively slow absorption. And its mortality rate is about 36 %. Pneumonia induced by H1N1 avian influenza virus is radiologically demonstrated as multiple flakes of ground glass opacity as well as patches and large flakes of high density consolidation, possibly with lobar or segmental atelectasis and pleural effusion. And its mortality rate is about 6 %.

Case 2

[Brief Medical History]

A 26-year-old woman, being pregnant for more than 2 months, reported a history of fever since Feb. 11, 2006, with a body temperature of above 38.5 °C and the highest body temperature of up to 40 °C. She also experienced cough with a little phlegm as well as diarrhea early after onset. In a local hospital, routine blood test showed WBC count 6.1×10^9/L, GR% 74.9% and LY% 15.6%. Chest X-ray indicated pneumonia at the right lower lung. By physical examination, breathing sound at the right lower lung was low and no other obvious positive signs. On d 7 after onset, Feb. 18, 2006, she was transferred to another hospital due to persistent fever, aggravated cough with more phlegm, chest distress and difficulty breathing. By inquiries of her epidemiological history, she reported a definitive history of contact to sick/dead chicken in her home 7 days prior to the onset, Feb. 4, 2006. By routine blood test, WBC count 3.30×10^9/L, N 0.83, L 0.15 and PLT 56×10^9/L. Blood biochemistry showed AST 90U/L, CK 74U/L, and LDH 537U/L. By blood gas analysis, pH 7.426, PaO_2 25.1 mmHg, $PaCO_2$ 51 mmHg, HCO_3 19.4 mmol/, and SO_2% 92%. Respiratory secretions examination on d 9 after onset (specimens collected 1 day ago), Feb. 20, 2006, the virus nucleic acid positive for H5N1 avian influenza virus. By reexamination by national parallel laboratory, the finding was still positive, with H5N1 avian influenza virus isolation positive.

The patient experienced dyspnea and rapid progression on d 7 after onset, and the condition further progressed into ARDS on d 8 after onset. Because the simplex oxygen supplying therapy failed to maintain oxygenation, noninvasive mechanical ventilation was ordered on d 9 after onset to maintain continuous positive airway pressure (CPAP) with settings of 10 cm H_2O, FiO_2 45%, and an elevated SaO_2 to 90–93%. But the noninvasive mechanical ventilation was discontinued due to shortness of breath and frequent cough of the patient. Subsequently, invasive nasotracheal intubation for ventilation was performed on that day. Tracheotomy was then performed for invasive ventilation 3 days after nasotracheal intubation.

On d 10 after onset, her body temperature returned to normal, but on d 14 after onset, the body temperature rose again to 37.5 °C, with increased peripheral hemogram and yellowish purulent bronchial secretions. A diagnosis of secondary bacterial infection was made and the administered antibiotics were adjusted accordingly. On d 16 after onset, miscarriage occurred. And on d 18 after onset, the invasive ventilation was discontinued, which was given for 10 days. On d 21 after onset, tracheal extubation was performed. And on d 20 after onset, her hemogram returned to normal indicating controlled secondary infection and convalescent stage of the disease. On Mar. 23, 2006 (d 40 after onset), the patient was discharged according to the criteria in Clinical Guidelines for Human Infected Avian Influenza (revised version, 2005) formulated by Ministry of Health, P. R. China.

[Radiological demonstration] Fig. 10.2.

[Diagnosis] Human infected H5N1 avian influenza.

[Discussion]

The patient is characterized by young woman, contact to sick/dead chicken 7 days before onset, initial symptom of fever, and normal WBC count. Her condition rapidly developed into pneumonia within 1 week after onset, and further rapidly into respiratory failure and multiple organs dysfunction.

Chest X-ray showed early exudation opacity in the right lower lung (d 4 after onset), and exudation opacity in bilateral middle and lower lung fields (d 6 after onset). On d 11 after onset, chest X-ray showed the most serious conditions, with large consolidation opacity in the right lung and the left middle lung. On d 12 after onset, oxygenation was improved, but slow absorption of the lesions was revealed by both chest X-ray and chest CT scan. On discharge, chest CT scan still demonstrated extensive spots, flakes and cords like opacity in both lungs.

The case is special in the following aspects:

1. Rapid progression of the condition.

   On d 6 after onset, chest X-ray demonstrated obvious deterioration of lesions every 3 h. Clinically, the patient experienced dyspnea and blood gas analysis indicated respiratory failure.
2. Pregnancy.

   At the onset of the symptoms, the patient was pregnant for more than 2 months and miscarriage occurred on d 16 after onset, which was within the expectation of the physicians. Complete curettage of uterine cavity following intraveneous anesthesia was successfully performed to remove fetus and placenta.
3. Blood gas analysis and chest X-ray.

   On d 12 after onset, blood gas analysis, routine blood test and biochemical examination indicated improved condition of the patient. And on d 20 after onset, the above examinations indicated normal condition of the patient. However, chest X-ray and chest CT scan still demonstrated slow absorption of the consolidation opacity. On discharge, blood gas analysis indicated normal but chest CT scan demonstrated obvious pulmonary interstitial changes.

This case is one of the cured cases of human infected avian influenza, with comparatively severe condition and

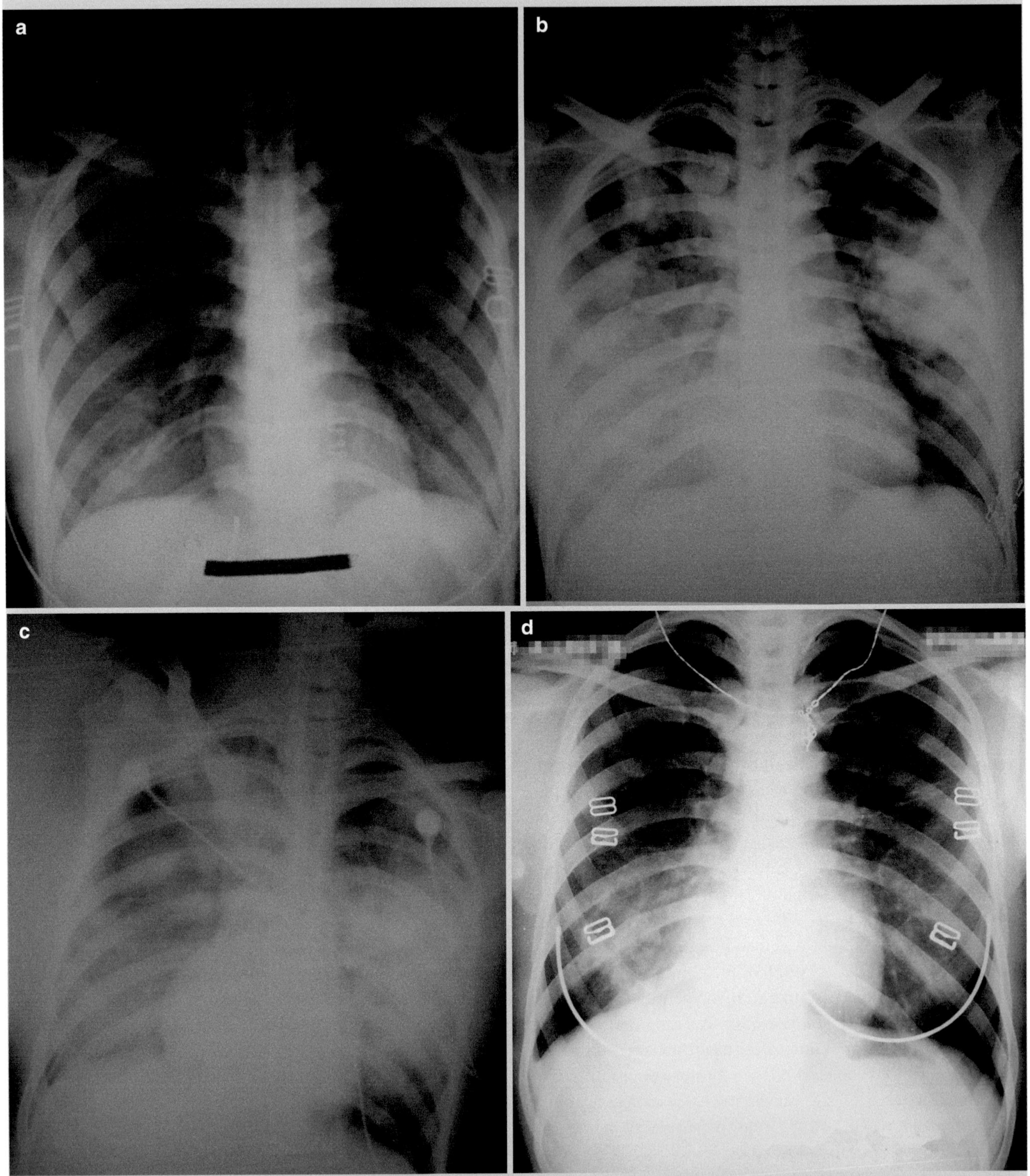

Fig. 10.2 (**a**) On d 4 after onset, chest X-ray demonstrated poorly defined flake of light opacity in the right lower lung field, and well defined left lung. (**b**) On d 7 after onset, the lesions were shown with rapid progression in a larger range in both lungs. Both lungs were shown with extensive cloudy and cotton like opacity and fusion of some into large flake. (**c**) On d 11 after onset, the lesions were shown to be within an even larger range in both lungs, namely the white-lung sign in both lungs, which indicated relapse and progression of the lesions. (**d**) On d 72 after onset, the both lungs were demonstrated with interstitial lesions, characterized by grid like opacity and obviously slower absorption. (**e**–**g**) On d 7 after onset, CT scan demonstrated extensive distribution of lesions in both lungs, which were more serious at the dorsal parts of both lungs, with air bronchogram in consolidation opacity. (**h**–**j**) On d 72 after onset, CT scan demonstrated obvious absorption of the lesions, cords like opacity in ground glass like change, and interlobular septal thickening in the peripheral areas of both lungs

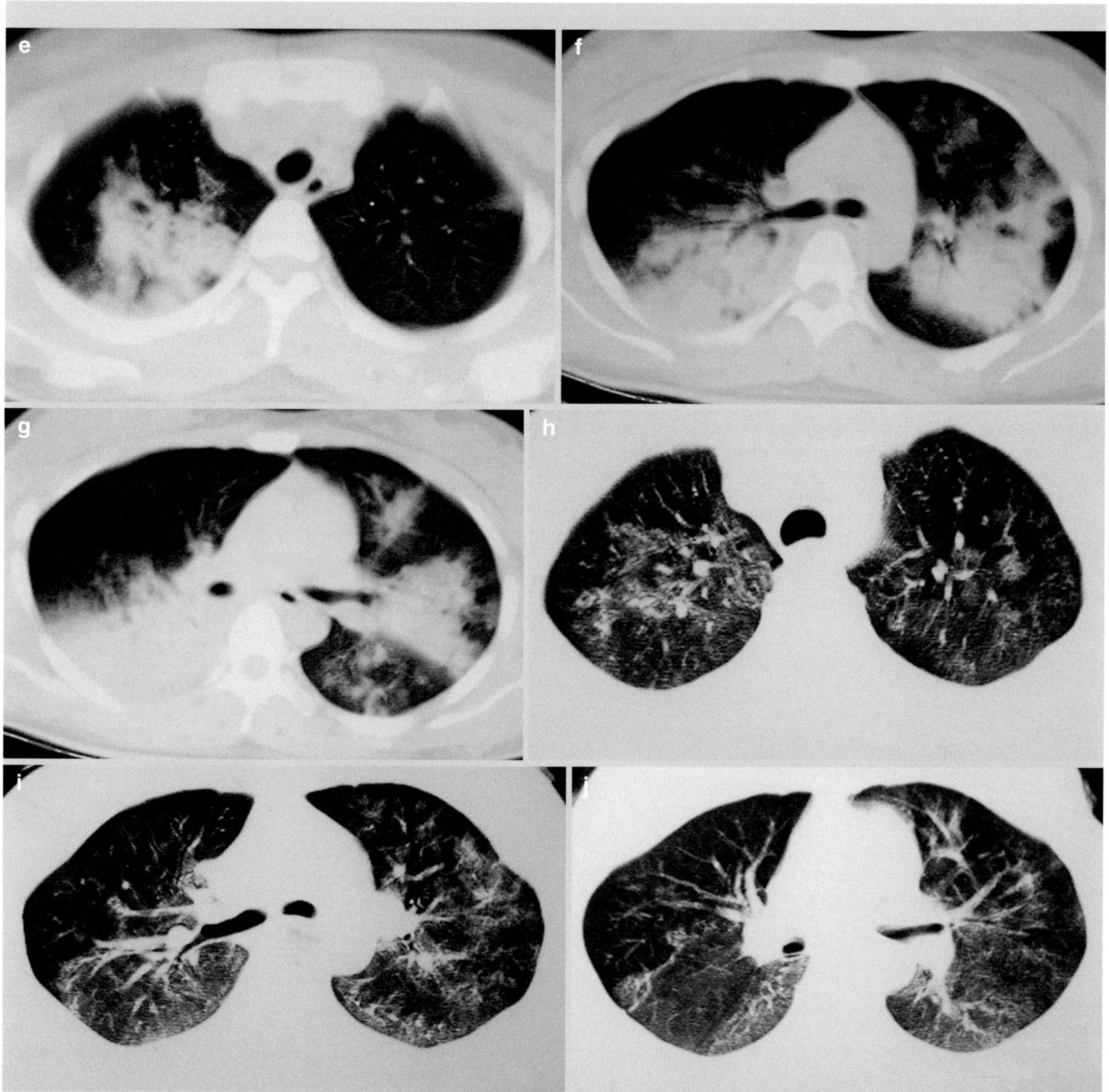

Fig. 10.2 (continued)

less complications. Only on d 14 after onset, the patient experienced re-elevated body temperature to 37.5 °C, with elevated peripheral hemogram and yellowish purulent bronchial secretions. The condition was diagnosed as secondary bacterial infection and the administered antibiotics were adjusted accordingly. On d 20 after onset, the hemogram returned to normal, indicating controlled secondary infection and convalescent stage of the disease. After her discharge, her serum collected at the convalescent stage was collaboratively administered to cure a patient with human infected H5N1 avian influenza in Shenzhen, Guangdong, China, which is known as the patient with the most serious condition among patients with H5N1 avian influenza.

By radiology, the key points for differential diagnosis are as the following:

Based on early chest CT scan, the lesions are demonstrated as poorly defined large flakes of increased density opacity, which are bilaterally symmetric. In combination to the clinical symptoms of high fever and cough, it should be differentiated from bacterial pneumonia of both lungs. However, the patient reported a history of contact, with normal level of peripheral WBC count. By dynamic observations via radiological examination, the lesions in both lungs progressed rapidly, with extensive involvement in bilateral lung fields and concurrent ground glass opacity and pulmonary consolidation opacity. All of these manifestations and findings are in consistency with pneumonia induced by human infected avian influenza. In addition, pneumonia induced by highly pathogenic H5N1 avian influenza virus should also be differentiated from SARS, AIDS complicated by PCP, and pneumonia induced by H7N9 avian influenza virus. Further differentiation should be comprehensively based on epidemiological history, etiological examination, clinical manifestations, and radiological findings.

References

Lu PX, Zhou BP. Clinical imaging diagnosis of emerging infectious diseases. Beijing: People's Medical Publishing House; 2013.

Lu PX, Zhou BP, Zhu WK, et al. Radiological demonstrations of pneumonia induced by highly pathogenic H5N1 avian influenza virus. Chin J Med Imaging Technol. 2007a;23(4):532–5.

Lu PX, Zhu WK, Ye RX, et al. CT demonstrations and their dynamic changes in adult patients with severe pneumonia induced by H5N1 avian influenza virus. Chin J CT MRI. 2007b;5(1):31–4.

Lu PX, Wang PX, Zhou BP, et al. Radiological features of lung changes caused by avian influenza subtype A H5N1 virus: report of two severe adult cases with regular follow-up. Chin Med J (Engl). 2010;123(1):100–4.

Zhou BP, Li YM, Lu PX. Human infected avian influenza. Beijing: Science Press; 2007.

11 Human Infected H7N9 Avian Influenza

Yuxin Shi, Puxuan Lu, Yuxin Yang, Chunhong Hu, Haiying Jin, and Lili Kong

11.1 Introduction

11.1.1 Definition and Prevalence

Human infected H7N9 avian influenza is an acute respiratory infectious disease caused by subtype H7N9 of avian influenza virus. Since the first case was reported in Yangzi River Delta of China in Feb. 2013, the total cases with definitive diagnosis had been up to 451 cases, including 176 cases of death, by Dec. 31, 2014, with a mortality rate of roughly 39 %.

11.1.2 Epidemiology

11.1.2.1 Source of Infection

Currently, subtype H7N9 of avian influenza virus has been isolated from the secretions and excretions of poultry, which is highly homologous with human infected H7N9 avian influenza virus. The source of its infection may be poultry carrying H7N9 avian influenza virus. And no definite evidence has been found supporting interpersonal transmission of H7N9 avian influenza virus, but its limited continual transmission from person to person has not been excluded.

11.1.2.2 Route of Transmission

Human is infected via respiratory tract. And close contact to excretions or secretions of infected poultry and direct contact to the virus can also cause its infection.

11.1.2.3 Susceptible Population

Individuals who have a history of contact to poultry within 1 week prior to onset are high risk population, such as those engaging in poultry raising, selling, slaughtering and processing.

11.1.3 Clinical Manifestation

The patients commonly experience influenza like symptoms, such as fever, cough with a little sputum, accompanying headache, muscle soreness and general malaise. In severe cases, the condition rapidly progresses, commonly into severe pneumonia within 5–7 days and the body temperature mostly above 39 °C, with dyspnea and accompanying bloody sputum. The condition may rapidly develop into acute respiratory distress syndrome (ARDS), sepsis, septic shock, and even multiple organs failure. Some patients may also develop mediastinal emphysema and pleural effusion. And its incubation period generally lasts for no more than 7 days.

11.1.4 Laboratory Test

11.1.4.1 Routine Blood Test

Generally, the WBC count may decrease. In severe cases, WBC count and lymphocyte count commonly decrease, possibly with decreased platelets.

Y. Shi (✉)
Affiliated Clinical Center of Public Health, Fudan University, Shanghai, China
e-mail: shiyx828288@163.com

P. Lu
Affiliated Shenzhen Third People's Hospital, Guangdong Medical College, Shenzhen, Guangdong, China

Y. Yang
Xinjiang Sixth People's Hospital, Urumuqi, Xinjiang, China

C. Hu
Affiliated First Hospital, Suzhou University, Suzhou, Jiangsu, China

H. Jin
Affiliated Huaihe Hospital, Henan University, Kaifeng, Henan, China

L. Kong
Yeda Hospital, Yantai, Shandong, China

H. Li (ed.), *Radiology of Influenza*, DOI 10.1007/978-94-024-0908-6_11

11.1.4.2 Blood Biochemistry

By blood biochemistry, the levels of creatine kinase, lactic dehydrogenase, aspartate amino transferase, alanine aminotransferase show increases. And C reactive protein level increases, possibly with increase of myohemoglobin level.

11.1.4.3 Etiological and Related Examination

Before anti-viral therapy is prescribed, it is necessary to collect the respiratory secretions for examination, such as nasopharyngeal secretions, oral gargle, tracheal aspirates or respiratory epithelial cells. In well equipped hospitals, the etiological examination should be performed immediately; while in poorly equipped hospitals, the specimen should be sent to entrusted institutions for etiological examination.

Antigen Screen of Influenza A Virus

Rapid detection for the antigen of influenza A virus in respiratory specimens can only be used for primary screening of human infected H7N9 avian influenza.

Nucleic Acid Test

PCR can be perform to examine respiratory secretions for subtype H7N9 of avian influenza virus.

Virus Isolation

The subtype H7N9 of avian influenza virus can be isolated from specimens of respiratory secretions.

Dynamic Detection of Paired Sera

In the patients with human infected H7N9 avian influenza virus, the specific antibody of H7N9 avian influenza virus increases at least 4 times.

11.1.5 Chest Radiology

Clinically, human infected H7N9 avian influenza can be categorized into 3 types, namely asymptomatic (latent infection), slight and severe. In the hospital we work in, 18 patients were hospitalized, with 1 case of slight infection and 17 cases of severe infection. The patient with slight infection only experienced flue like symptoms, such as fever, but no lung abnormality. However, the 17 patients with severe infection experienced severe pneumonia, with the conditions meeting the diagnostic criteria of severe pneumonia induced by H7N9 avian influenza virus issued by National Health and Family Planning Commission. The clinical manifestations of severe pneumonia induced by human infected H7N9 avian influenza are as the following:

11.1.5.1 Early Stage

The early lesions are mainly located in lower lobe of one lung, predominantly with a segmental distribution. Radiologically, they are ground glass opacity, interlobular septal thickening and acinar nodules.

11.1.5.2 Progressive Stage

The pulmonary lesions progresses rapidly from small flakes of opacity to large consolidations, from one segment to multiple segments, from one lung to both lungs, and from lower lobes to the whole lungs. Within 24–48 h, the pulmonary lesions may spread rapidly to involve multiple lobes of both lungs. In severe cases, the pulmonary lesions show a significant increase ($\geq 50\%$) within several hours. The lesions develop rapidly from ground glass opacity to consolidation opacity, and the density of consolidation opacity increases, with occurrence of serous effusion. The pulmonary lesions commonly reach their peak within 5–0 days, with observable lung air sac at this time.

11.1.5.3 Convalescent Stage

For the cases with no complication, if prompt anti-viral therapy administered, the lesions begin to be absorbed slowly after their reaching the peak, firstly the ground glass opacity, and then consolidations and the lesions in the central area adjacent to the hilum. The consolidations show decreasing density to sparse and the consolidated lung tissues gradually inflate. During the whole process of absorption, the lesions in middle and upper lung lobes are absorbed earlier than the lesions in dorsal lower lung lobes and the subpleural lesions. The early lesions that emerge during the early and progressive stages are absorbed late, and the lesions that emerge late are firstly absorbed. Radiologically, pulmonary fibrosis is demonstrated as small patches, fibrous cords like, grid like, and small ground glass opacity in subpleural areas of both lungs and/or doral segments of both lower lungs. Meanwhile, subpleural paraseptal emphysema, scar type emphysema, subpleual lung bullae and limited bronchiectasis are revealed.

11.2 Typical Cases

Case 1

[Brief Case History]

A 53-year-old man of Han nationality complained of intermittent fever for 13 days and difficulty breathing for 4 days that aggravated as well as unconsciousness for 2 h. After ineffective treatment in another hospital, he was transferred to our hospital on Aug. 16, 2014. Laboratory tests showed nucleic acid of H7N9 avian influenza virus positive, with increased neutrophils and decreased lymphocytes. Blood biochemistry revealed increased levels of γ-glutamyl transpeptidase, lactate dehydrogenase and α-hydrobutyrate dehydrogenase. During hospitalization for treatment, he received bed-side chest DR radiography per day (totally 8 bed-side chest DR films and 3 chest CT scans) to assess his conditions. After emergency rescuing, he was cured and discharged on Sep. 5, 2014. After that, he received 2 follow-up chest CT scans for re-examination.

[Radiological demonstration] Fig. 11.1

[Diagnosis] Pneumonia induced by human infected H7N9 avian influenza virus, severe pneumonia, and ARDS.

[Discussion]

Pneumonia induced by human infected H7N9 avian influenza is an acute respiratory infectious disease caused by subtype H7N9 of avian influenza virus and it occurs in any age group of people. Before onset, the patient usually has a history of exposure to an environment contaminated by avian influenza virus, and the common clinical manifestations include cough, expectoration, and fever. The condition progresses rapidly in seriously ill patients, with occurrence of severe pneumonia within 3–7 days after onset. The body temperature mostly persists above 39 °C with dyspnea, which rapidly further progresses into acute respiratory distress syndrome (ARDS), sepsis, septic shock, and even multiple organs failure.

Pneumonia induced by human infected H7N9 avian influenza is radiologically characterized by the following:

1. Morphologically, the lesions are pulmonary consolidation, ground glass opacity and interstitial changes.
2. The lesions are diffusely distributed in both lungs in severe cases, which are more serious in lower lungs.
3. The lesions show rapid progression, with emergence or increase of consolidations during the progressive stage.
4. The primary ground glass opacity in lungs shows obvious consolidation inside within a short period of time. Otherwise, the range with primary consolidations enlarges with increased density.
5. The lesions are migratory, with absorption of primary lesions within a short period of time and newly emerging lesions in other parts of lungs, which are radiologically characteristic.
6. The lesions show slow absorption, with signs of pulmonary fibrosis after cured.
7. Chest CT demonstrations are inconsistent to the clinical symptoms because the absorption of lesions lags behind. Re-examination by chest CT scan show slight absorption of the lung lesions after the clinical symptoms are obviously improved.

Pneumonia induced by human infected H7N9 avian influenza should be differentiated from the following diseases:

1. Pneumonia induced by influenza virus
   Its occurrence is related to prevalence of influenza, with rapid progression. Radiologically, the lesions are mainly confined and segmental alveolar consolidation, which may further develop into diffuse lesions with air bronchogram. By chest X-ray, it shares commonalities with pneumonia induced by H7N9 avian influenza, and their differential diagnosis is challenging. And its final definitive diagnosis should be based on the laboratory tests.
2. Adenoviral pneumonia
   It is more common in children whose chest X-ray demonstrations include increased, thickened and blurry lung markings. The lesions distribute extensively,

Fig. 11.1 Chest X-ray demonstrated consolidation and ground glass opacity in the right upper lung and the left lower lung, with uneven density, poorly defined boundary, and inner air bronchogram (**a**). Re-examination after 4 days demonstrated consolidation and ground glass opacity in the right upper lung and the left lower lung, with decreased density and smaller lesion range (**b**). Re-examination after 6 days showed consolidation and ground glass opacity in the right upper lung and the left lower lung, with further decreased density and smaller lesion range (**c**). Re-examination after 12 days revealed consolidation and ground glass opacity in the right upper lung and the left lower lung, with further decreased density and smaller lesion range; and partially interstitial fibrosis (**d**). Re-examination by chest CT scan after 36 days demonstrated multiple small patches of dense opacity in both lungs and in lateral part of lungs, predominantly in the right upper lung and the left lower lung, and partially interstitial fibrosis (**e**, **f**). Re-examination by chest CT scan after 5 months demonstrated obviously decreased small patches of dense opacity in both lungs, with rare fibrous cords like opacity (**g**)

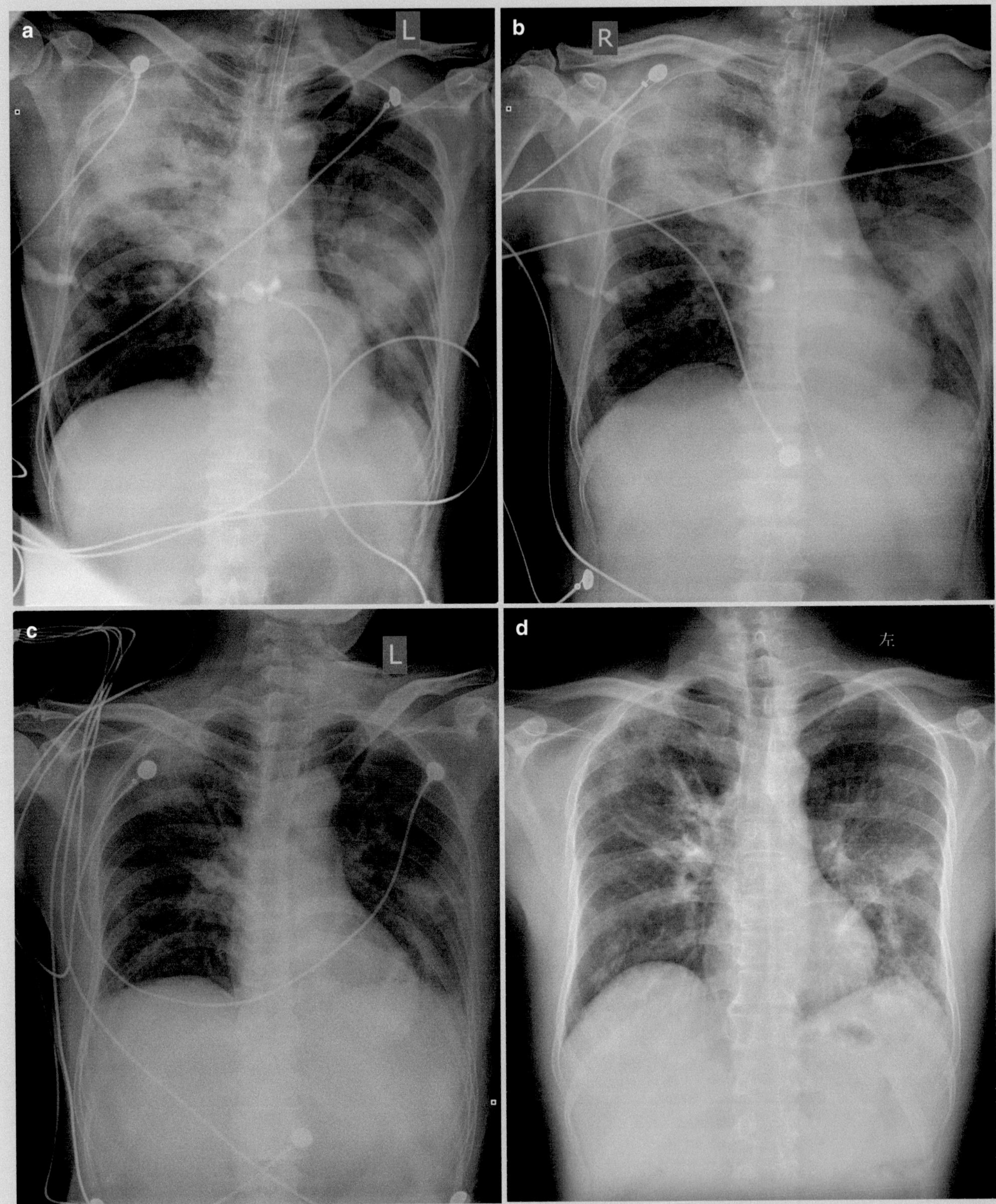

Fig. 11.1 (continued)

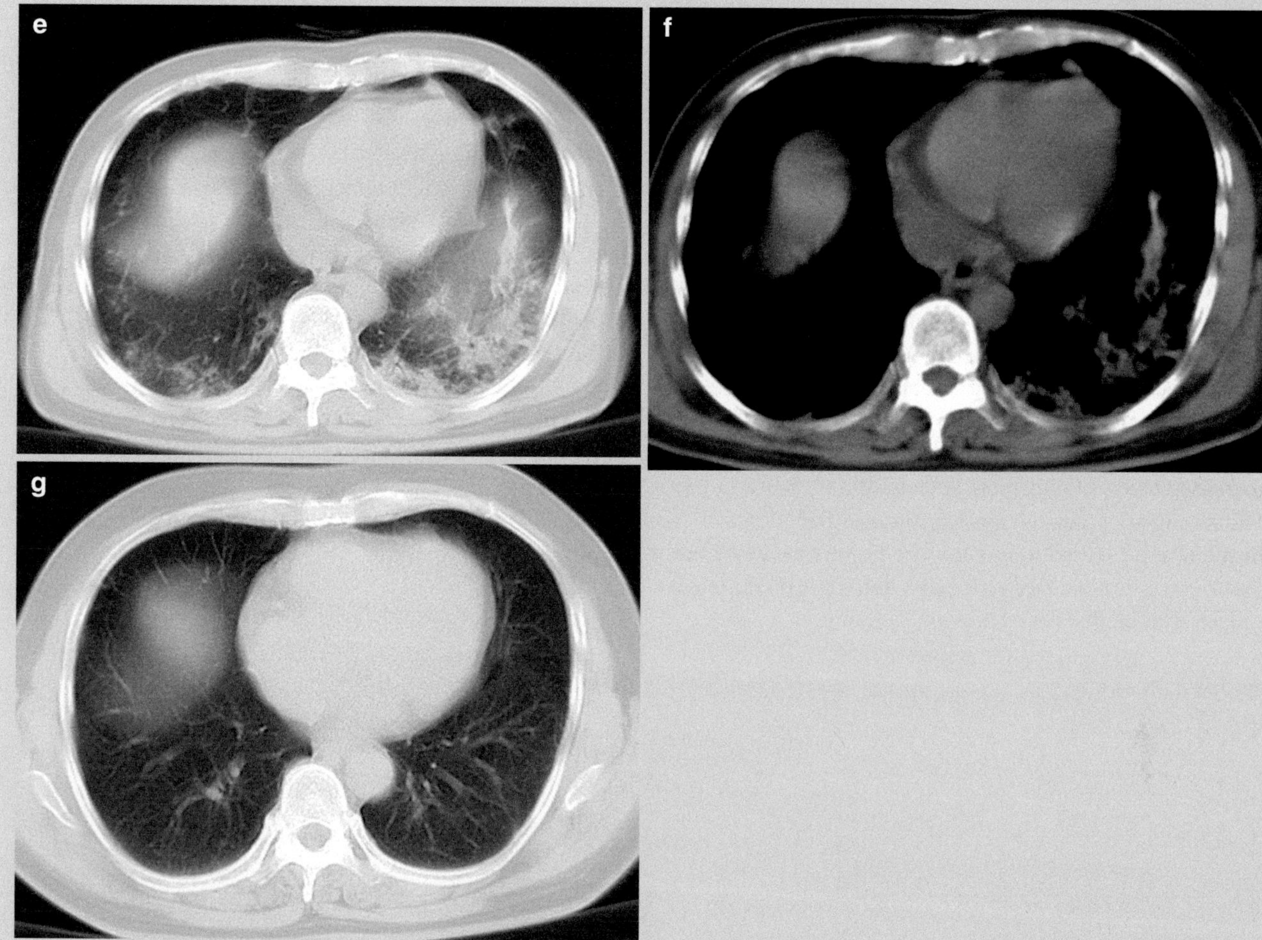

Fig. 11.1 (continued)

which are characterized by many lung markings, many lesions of emphysema, many integrated lesions and many large lesions, but rare round lesions, rare lesions of lung bullae and rare pleural effusion as well as consistency between radiological signs and clinical symptoms.

3. Severe acute respiratory syndrome (SARS)
   The patients with SARS have definite epidemiological history of contact. By chest X-ray, it is demonstrated with diversifying lesions, among which cotton like exudation is the most common; multi-focus granuloma and false cavity are possibly its specific signs.

Case 2

[Brief Case History]

A 65-year-old man of Han Chinese, experienced cough, expectoration, obvious increase of the body temperature, dyspnea, tachypnea, chest distress and shortness of breath. By CT scan in another hospital, inflammation of both lungs and bilateral pleural effusion were revealed. He was transferred into our hospital on Dec. 12, 2014. Laboratory tests showed the nucleic acid of H7N9 avian influenza virus positive; eutrophils within normal range, decreased lymphocytes count; increased levels of γ-glutamyl transpeptidase, lactate dehydrogenase, α-hydrobutyrate dehydrogenase, serum lipoprotein, and C reactive protein; increased creatinine level that exceeded the normal range as well as increased levels of creatinine and cystatin C. Bedside chest DR radiography per day (totally 5 chest DR films) in our hospital was ordered to monitor the lesion changes. Death finally occurred on Dec. 16, 2014 due to multiple organs failure after ineffective emergency rescuing.

[Radiological demonstration] Fig. 11.2

[Diagnosis] Critical case of human infected H7N9 avian influenza, severe pneumonia, ARDS, and multiple organs dysfunction.

[Discussion]

In this case, the patient was radiologically demonstrated with diffuse small patches of dense opacity in both lungs that are ground glass like as well as integration of lesions and enlarged range with lesions along with progression of the condition.

For this case, the condition should be differentiated from highly pathogenic H5N1 avian influenza, seasonal influenza (including type A influenza H1N1), bacterial pneumonia, SARS, novel coronaviral pneumonia, adenoviral pneumonia, chlamydia pneumonia, and mycoplasma pneumonia. The definitive diagnosis is mainly based on etiological examinations.

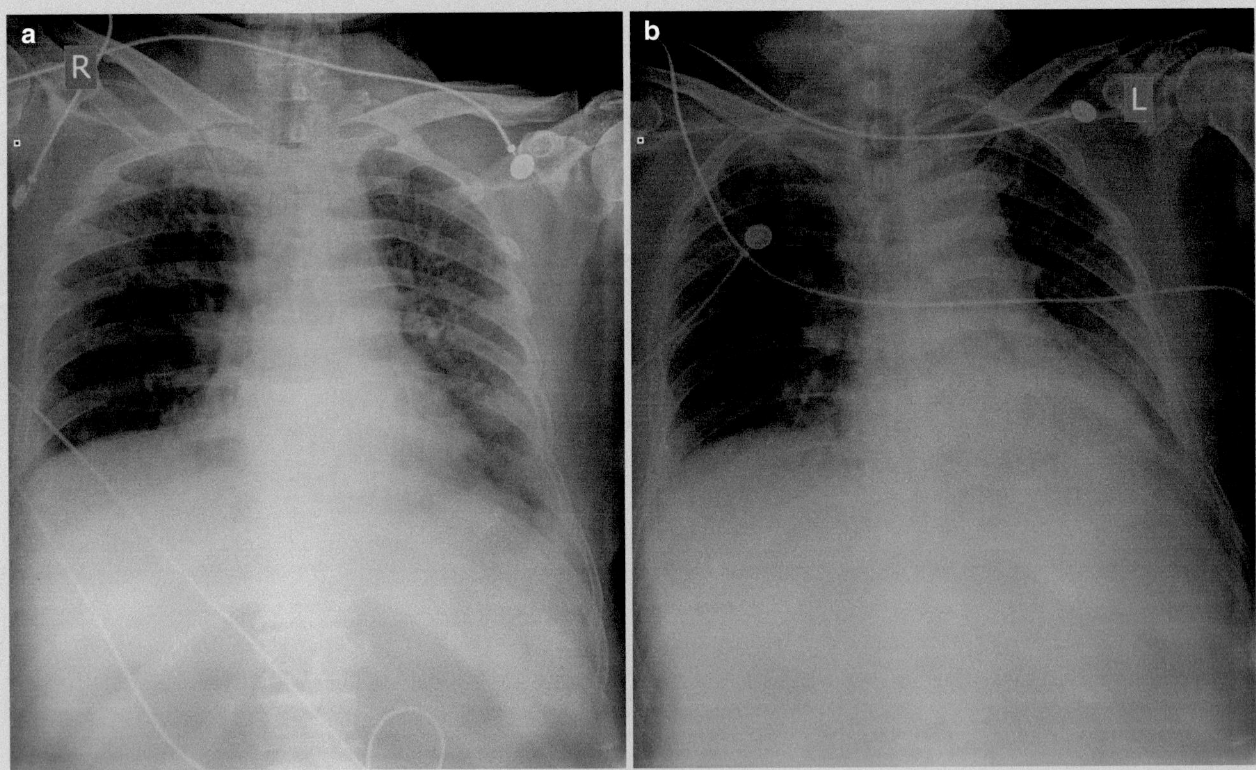

Fig. 11.2 Chest X-ray demonstrated diffuse small patches of dense opacity in both lungs that are ground glass like (**a**). Re-examination after 1 day showed diffuse small patches of dense opacity in both lungs that are ground glass like, with no obvious change compared to the previous chest X-ray (**b**). Re-examination after 3 days revealed diffuse small patches of dense opacity in both lungs that are ground glass like, some of which are integrated; enlarged range with lesions in the left lung and the right upper lung; increased density of the opacity (**c**). Re-examination after 4 days demonstrated diffuse small patches of dense opacity in both lungs that are ground glass like, with further aggravation (**d**)

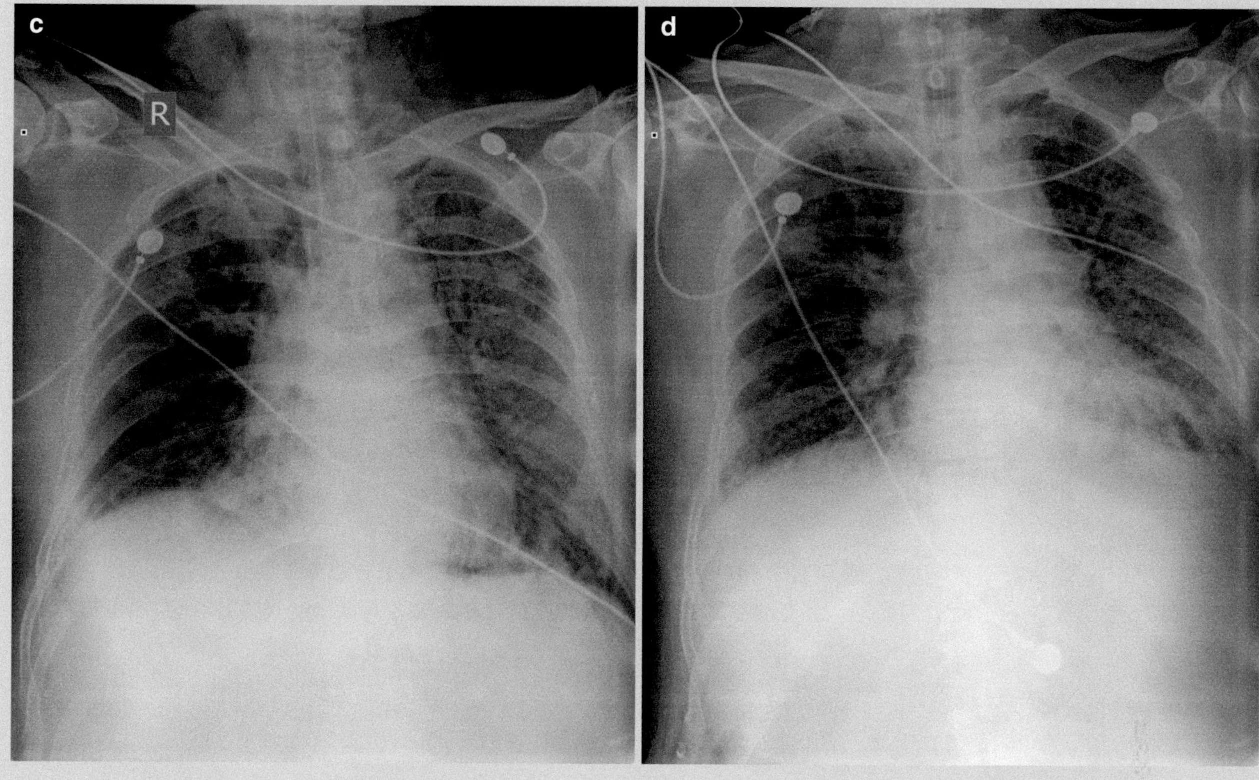

Fig. 11.2 (continued)

Case 3

[Brief Case History]

A 60-year-old man was hospitalized due to fever for 4 days and cough for 1 day. By physical examinations, his body temperature was 37.6 °C, with clear sound by lung percussion, clear breathing sounds by auscultation with no obvious dry and moist rales. Laboratory tests revealed WBC count 6.19×10^9/L, GR% 77.11 %, MONO% 12.4 %, lymphocytes ratio 10.32 %, hs-CRP 85 mg/L, and ESR 9 mm/h. Serological test for M. pneumoniae was negative and blood biochemistry showed no abnormity. Chest CT indicated large high-density opacity with uneven density and poorly defined boundary in the lingual segment of left upper lung lobe. And the diagnosis was considered to be pneumonia of the left lung. After treatment for 2 days, the patient still experienced fever and was transferred into a large hospital for treatment. After that, the patient showed persistent fever with a body temperature of 37.6 °C. Bedside chest X-ray after 10 days demonstrated increased and blurry lung markings and multiple cotton like and flakes of opacity in both lungs. Bedside color Doppler ultrasonography showed liquid opacity in the right thoracic cavity and pericardium. And the patient experienced continuous decrease of oxygen saturation to around 60 % and his blood pressure decreased to around 70/50 mmHg. At that night, throat swabs by professionals from CDC showed positive and the diagnosis was defined to be human infection of H7N9 avian influenza virus. The patient was then transferred to the local hospital specialized in infectious diseases, and death occurred 1 week later. The patient reported a history of close contacts to feces of birds and chickens.

[Radiological demonstration] Fig. 11.3

[Diagnosis] Pneumonia induced by human infected H7N9 avian influenza.

[Discussion]

Human infected H7N9 avian influenza is a type of type A influenza, with the first 3 cases reported in Shanghai and Anhui province of China in Mar. 2013. Human infected H7N9 avian influenza virus is a newly emerging recombinant virus, which infects human via respiratory tract after contact to poultry with the infection. It has an incubation period of no more than 7 days. And the patients commonly experience flu like symptoms, such as fever, cough, expectoration of a little sputum as well as accompanying headache, muscle soreness and general malaise. In severe cases, the condition progresses rapidly into severe pneumonia, mostly with a body temperature of above 39 °C, dyspnea and possibly accompanying bloody sputum. Severe pneumonia may further progresses rapidly into ARDS, mediastinal emphysema, sepsis, shock, consciousness disturbance, and acute renal damage. By chest radiology, the disease is characterized by primary lesions in one lung that gradually involve both lungs along with progression of the condition. In addition, the multiple lesions in both lungs show a multi-segmental and multi-lobar distribution. For this case, the patient had a history of close contacts to feces of birds, and the disease is radiologically characterized by inflammation of lobes in one lung at its early stage. Along with the progression of the condition, both lungs are rapidly involved and ARDS finally occurred. The diagnosis was defined based on the finding of throat swabs to be a typical case of human infected H7N9 avian influenza. For this case, the condition should be differentiated from other types of pneumonia. Compared to other types of pneumonia, the patient in this case showed no obvious characteristic symptoms and physical signs and the definitive diagnosis is mainly based on the etiological examination.

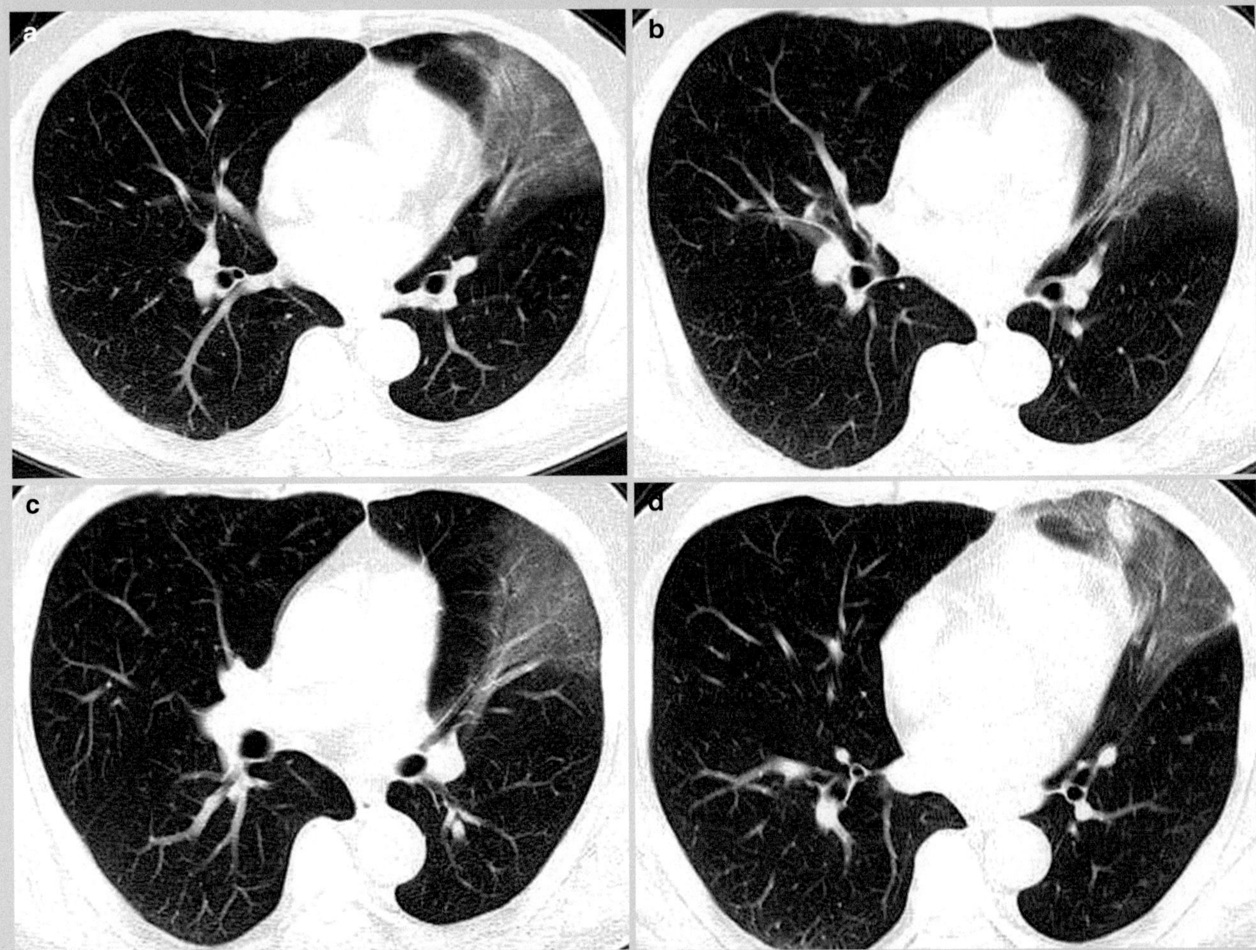

Fig. 11.3 CT scan demonstrated wedge shaped ground glass opacity in the lingual segment of left upper lung lobe, with high but uneven density, poorly defined boundary and air bronchogram inside (**a**–**d**)

Case 4

[Brief Case History]

A 20-year-old woman complained of fever with the highest body temperature of 39 °C, headache, cough, expectoration of rust colored sputum, and systemic malaise for 1 day. Laboratory test showed WBC 3.8 × 10^9/L. She denied a history of contact to poultry.

[Radiological demonstration] Fig. 11.4

[Diagnosis] Severe pneumonia induced by human infected H7N9 avian influenza.

[Discussion]

For this case, the chest radiology demonstrated:

1. In the early stage, chest X-ray demonstrated ground glass opacity in one lung that showed lobar distribution with no opacity across the interlobar fissure.
2. The lesions were predominantly ground glass opacity that rapidly progressed to involve both lungs, with diffuse distribution and enlarged range with lesions. The GGO was shown to develop into consolidations with air bronchogram inside.
3. After positive treatment, the lesions were gradually absorbed and improved, with smaller range with lesions, decreased density as well as evolvement into fibrous cords like, grid like and honeycomb like opacity.

Based on these radiological findings, we know that pneumonia induced by human infected H7N9 avian influenza resembles to other types of viral pneumonia, with concurrent parenchymal and interstitial involvements. However, pneumonia induced by human infected H7N9 avian influenza shows more obvious alveolar exudation in its early stage that overlaps lung interstitium. After partial absorption of alveolar exudation, fibrous cords like, grid like and honeycomb like opacity are radiologically demonstrated.

In this case, the condition should be differentiated from bacterial pneumonia and pneumonia induced by H1N1 influenza. By radiology, bacterial pneumonia is characterized by increased and blurry lung markings and nonspecific patchy opacity in both lungs, which is more common in bilateral middle and lower lung fields as well as middle and medial parts of both lungs. Clinically, WBC count increases. Pneumonia induced by H1N1 influenza shows early signs of GGO lesions in subpleural area and around bronchi. For this case, the differential diagnosis is challenging and should be based on virological detection.

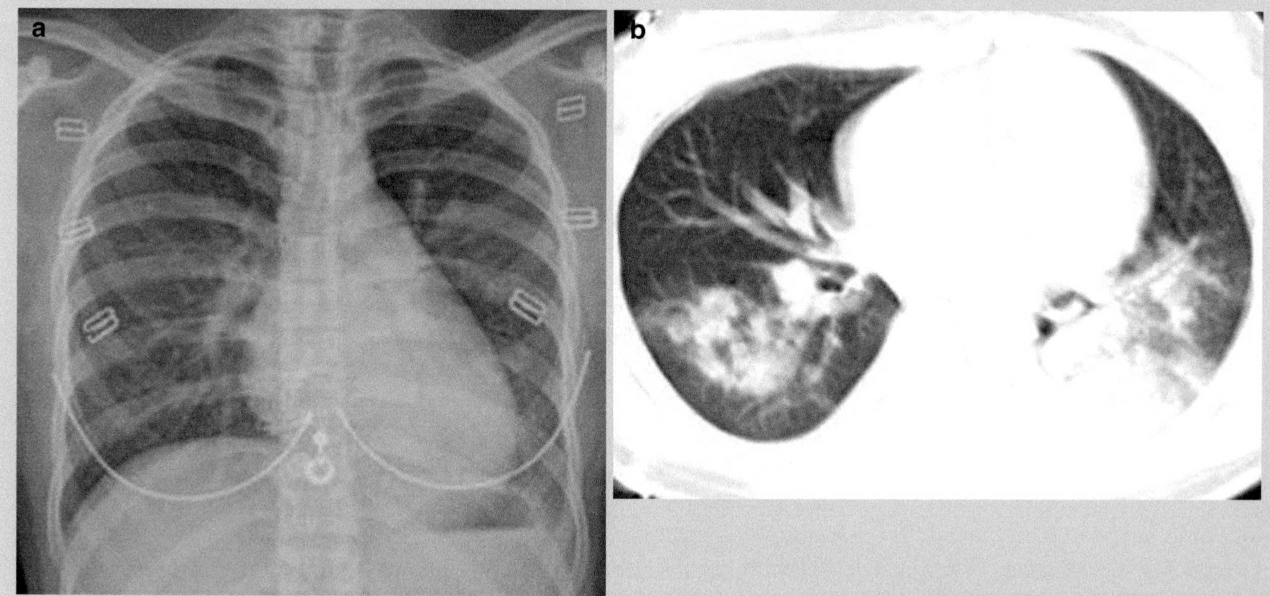

Fig. 11.4 Anterior-posterior chest x-ray 1 day after onset showed increased and thickened lung markings; small ground glass opacity in the left upper lung (**a**). Chest CT on d 3 after onset showed multiple patchy and nodular consolidations in both lungs, predominantly in the lower lung (**b**). Re-examination CT scan on d 5 after onset showed progression of the lesions into large consolidation, with air bronchogram inside (**c**). Re-examination after anti-viral treatment on d 9 after onset showed obvious absorption of pulmonary lesions, with smaller range with lesions and decreased density (**d**). Re-examination by CT scan on d 12 showed further absorption of the lesions (**e**). Re-examination by CT scan on d 23 after onset showed fibrous cords like and honeycomb like opacity in both lungs (**f**)

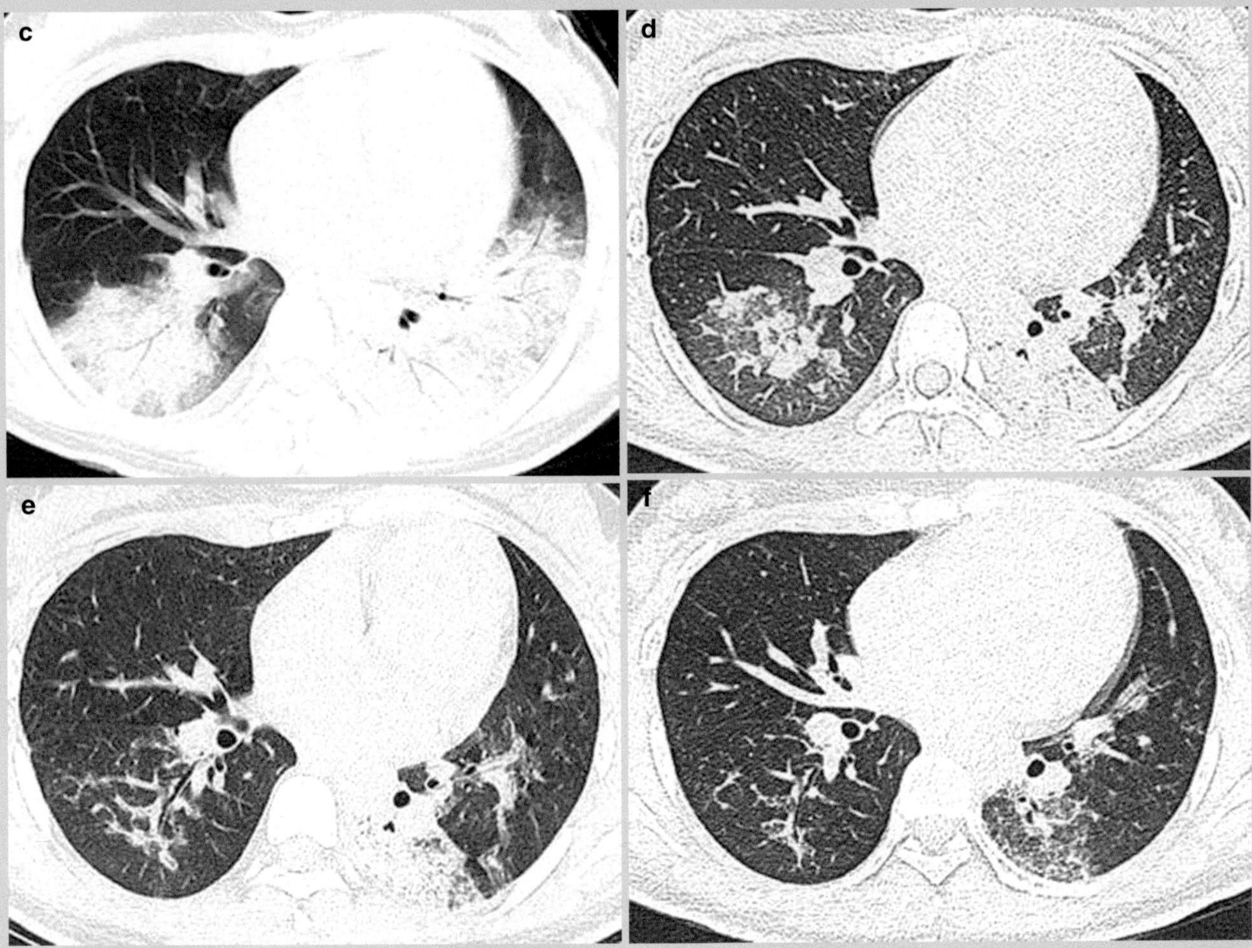

Fig. 11.4 (continued)

Case 5

[Brief Case History]

A 79-year-old woman experienced nasal obstruction, runny nose, fever with the highest body temperature of 39 °C, cough and expectoration. She denied a recent history of contact to poultry and denied a history of contact to patient with influenza. She was detected with nucleic acid of H7N9 avian influenza virus positive. Sputum culture revealed A. baumanii positive (++++) and aspergillosis positive. She had a medical history of cholestatic hepatocirrhosis as well as coronary heart disease and atrial fibrillation for 10 years. And she had medical history of right femoral neck fracture 4 months ago due to traumatic injury, which was treated by internal fixation and replacement. Currently, she was bedridden for a long period of time, and death finally occurred.

[Radiological demonstration] Fig. 11.5

[Diagnosis] Pneumonia induced by H7N9 avian influenza, Mixed lung infection by Aspergillus and A. baumanii.

[Discussion]

Recently, literature reports indicated that the susceptible populations to pneumonia induced by human infected H7N9 avian influenza include the elderly, those with underlying disease or compromised immunity. By CT scans, the most common sign is ground glass opacity, followed by consolidation, air bronchogram and interlobular septal thickening. The condition may be complicated by pleural effusion or air containing cyst. The lesions of the disease show a wide range, commonly involving 3 or more lung lobes. Qingle et al. reported a group of cases, with no formation of cavity. For this case, the patient was an elderly, with medical histories of hepatocirrhosis, femoral neck fracture, long-term bedridden and compromised immunity. By sputum culture, Aspergillus was positive, indicating a complication of pulmonary aspergillosis, which is most likely the reason for intrapulmonary nodules and cavities. In addition, she also showed an infection of A. baumanii and death finally occurred. All the above clinical symptoms and radiological signs indicated that pneumonia induced by H7N9 avian influenza may be further complicated by fungal and bacterial infection, particularly in the elderly patients with poor condition of health and compromised immunity.

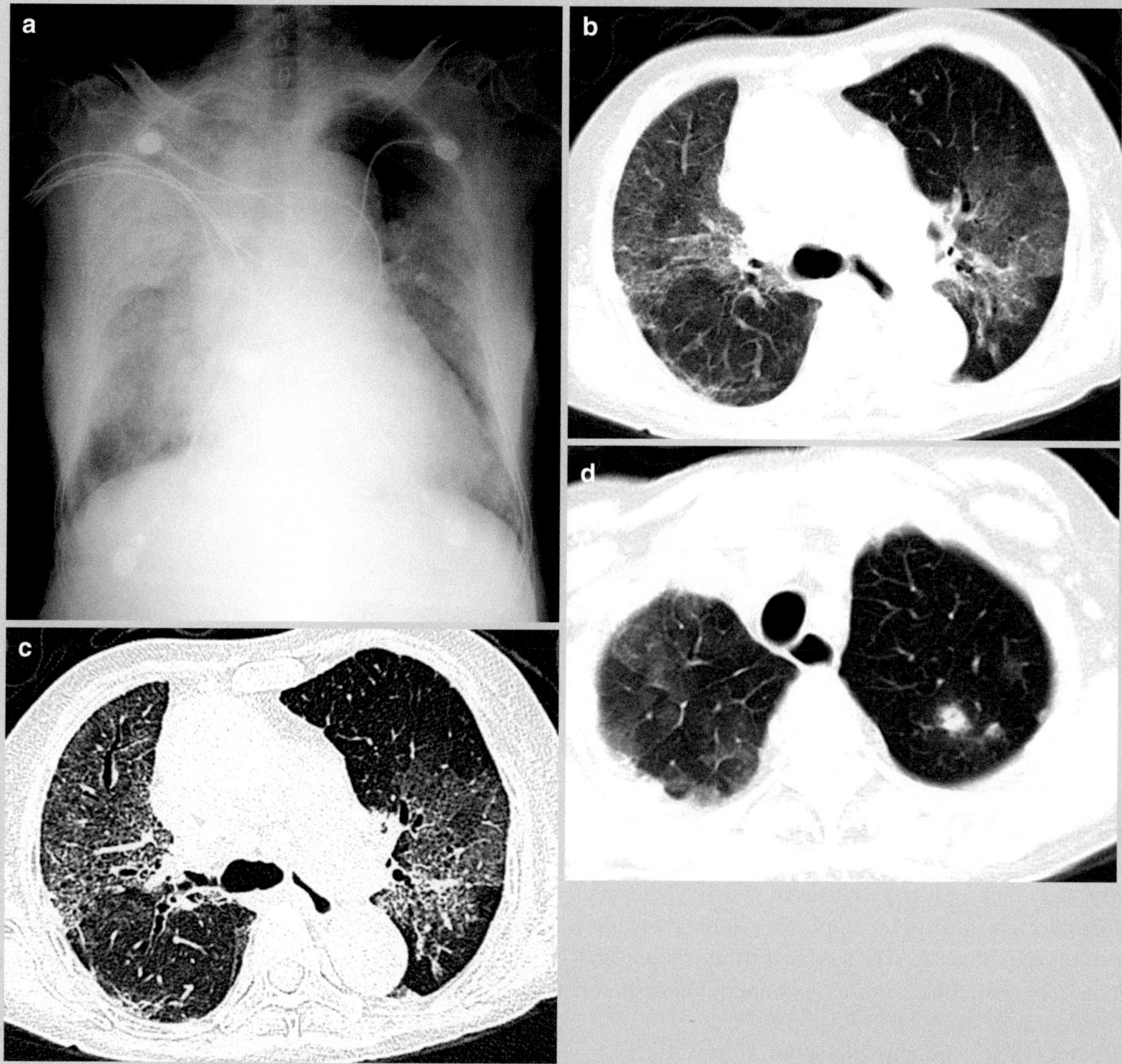

Fig. 11.5 Bedside chest X-ray demonstrated decreased transparency of both lungs, with diffuse large high density opacity that was more obvious in the right lung than in the left lung (**a**). CT scan showed diffuse ground glass opacity, grid like opacity, and flakes of high density opacity in both lungs; nodular opacity in the left upper lung lobe and in the right middle lung lobe; halo signs around the nodules in the left upper lung lobe (**c** was the 1 mm reconstructed image of the same layer as **b**) (**b**–**e**). Re-examination by CT scan after 2 days showed no improvement of the lung lesions; cavity within the nodules in the left upper lung; halo sign around the nodules; obviously enlarged nodules in the right middle lung lobe (**f**, **g**)

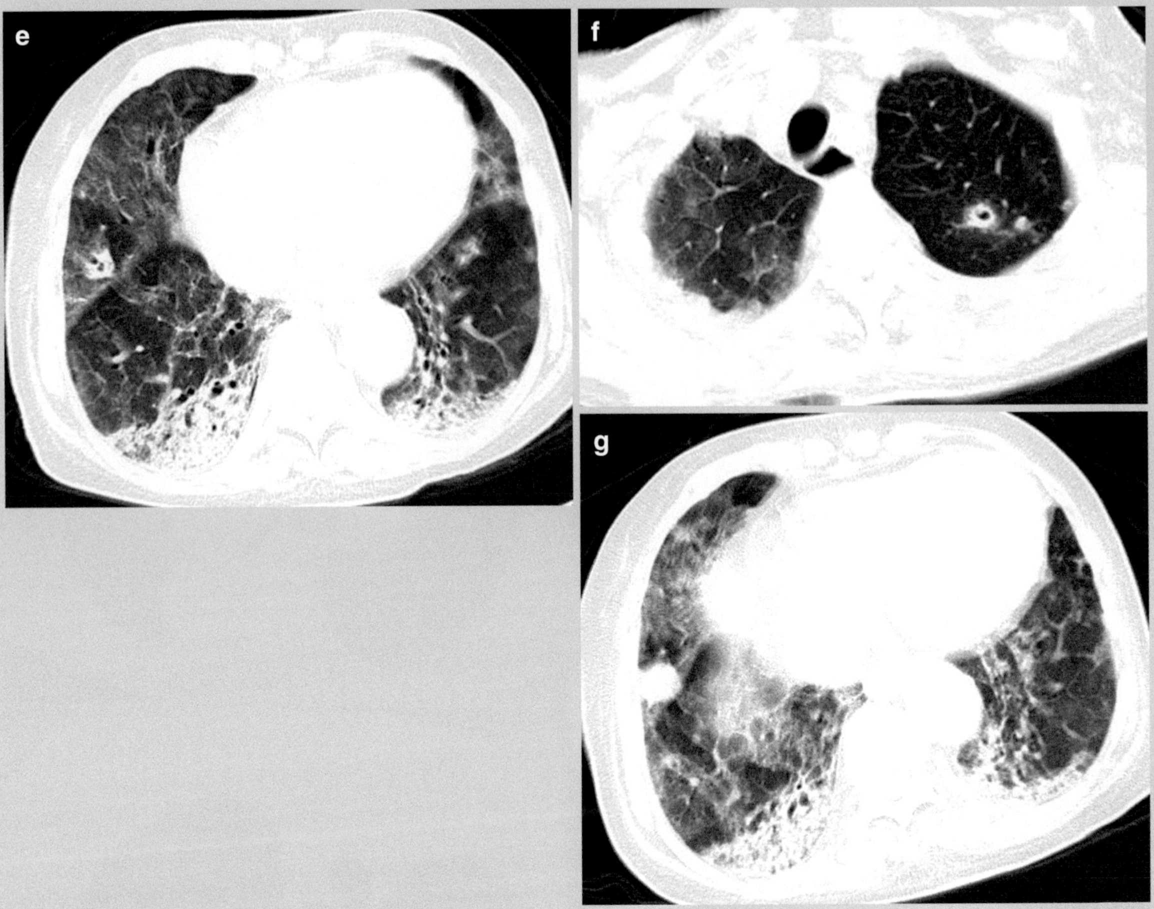

Fig. 11.5 (continued)

Case 6

[Brief Case History]

A 67-year-old man experienced fever, cough, and expectoration of a little whitish sputum, with the highest body temperature of 38.5 °C. He has no history of physical examination and other histories of underlying diseases. The nucleic acid test for H7N9 was positive.

[Radiological demonstration] Fig. 11.6

[Diagnosis] Pneumonia induced by human infected H7N9 avian influenza.

[Discussion]

The most common sign of pneumonia induced by human infected H7N9 avian influenza by CT scan is ground glass opacity, followed by consolidation, air bronchogram and interlobular septal thickening, possibly with pleural effusion. In some cases, air containing cyst can be observed, with a large area of involvement, commonly 3 or even more lung lobes. During the treatment, the condition may repeatedly improve and deteriorate, with the lung lesions firstly absorbed and then progress that is rapid in some cases. In some patients with good physical constitution and early diagnosis, the condition can be obviously improved after several days treatment, just like the present case. By CT scan, pneumonia induced by human infected H7N9 avian influenza is demonstrated with no specific signs, resembling to other viral pneumonia. And the final diagnosis should be based on clinical manifestations and laboratory tests. Radiological examinations play important role in guiding clinical treatment, monitoring disease progression, assessing therapeutic efficacy, and predicting the prognosis. Feng et al. scored the radiological demonstrations of pneumonia induced by human infected H7N9 avian influenza, which showed that a high score indicates a high mortality rate.

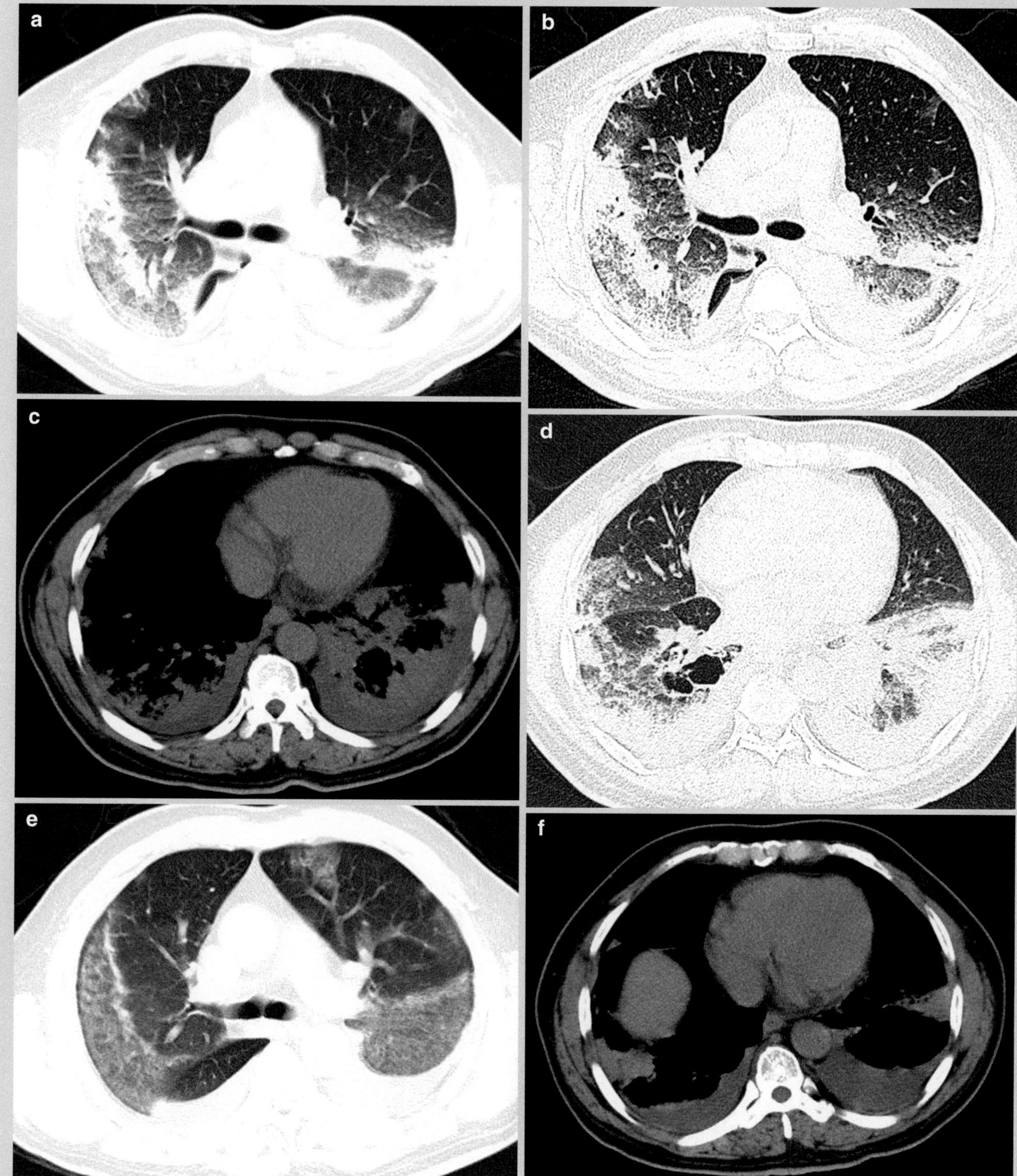

Fig. 11.6 CT scan showed multiple flakes of ground glass like and grid like high density opacities in both lungs, with air bronchogram within some lesions (**b** as the 1 mm reconstructed image of the same layer of **a**) (**a**, **b**). Bilateral pleural effusion in a small quantity (**c**). The basial segment of the right lower lung was shown with an irregular air containing cyst, with a little gas-fluid level (**d**). Reexamination after 4 days treatment, the lesions in the lungs were obviously absorbed (**e**). Bilateral pleural effusion progressed (**f**). The air containing cyst in the right lower lung showed no obvious changes (**g**). Re-examination after 1 month, the lesions in lungs were obviously absorbed, still with flakes and grid like high density opacity that predominantly under the pleura (**i** as the 1 mm reconstructed image of the same layer of **h**) (**h**, **i**). Bilateral pleural effusion was completely absorbed. (**j**) The air containing cyst in the right lower lung was enlarged (**k**)

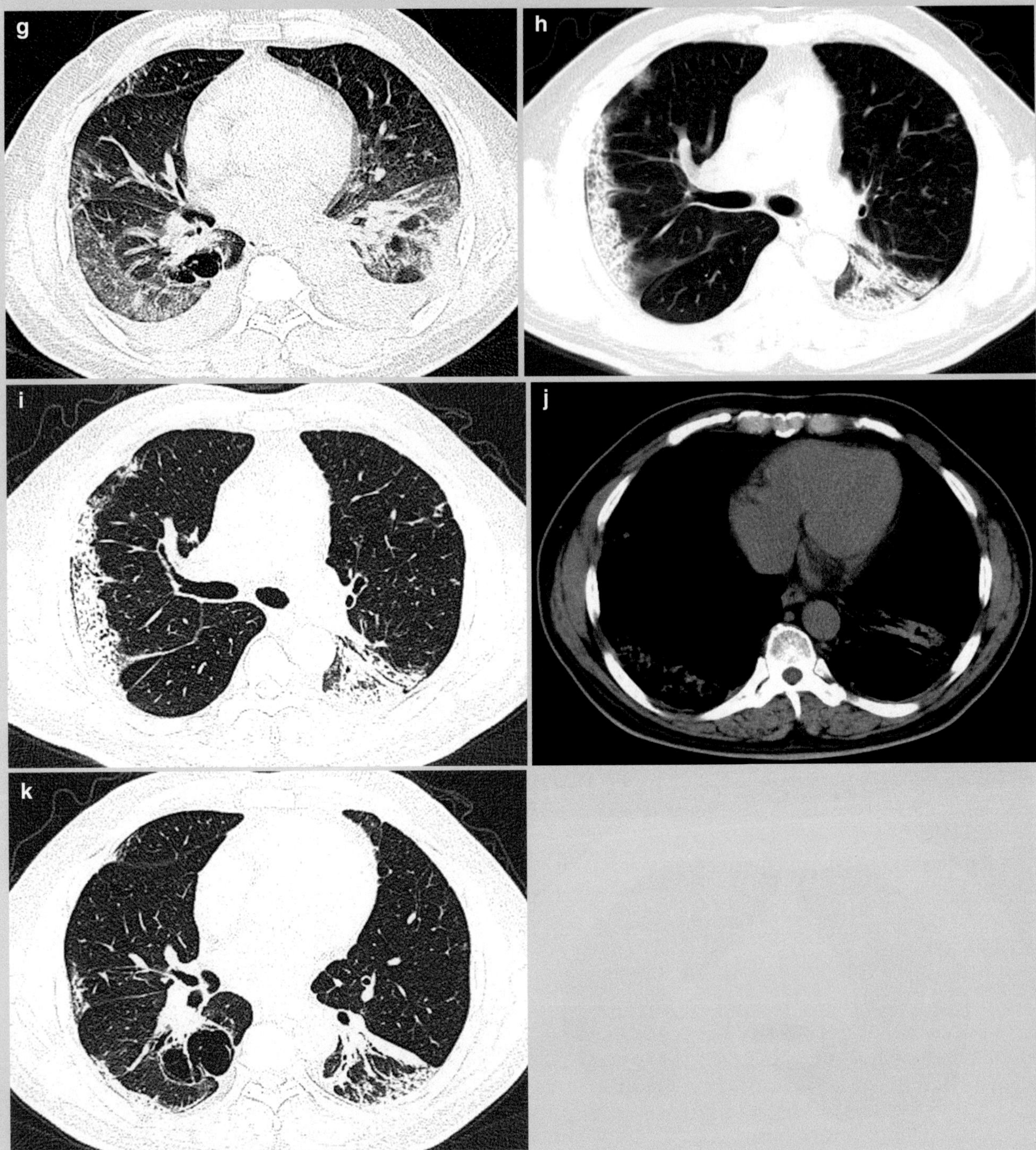

Fig. 11.6 (continued)

Case 7

[Brief Case History]

A 33-year-old man, working as a cook, was hospitalized due to the chief complaints of chest distress for 5 days that deteriorated, with fever, cough and expectoration for 3 days. About 5 days ago, the patient caught a cold and began to experience chest distress that deteriorated after physical activities, and the body temperature within normal limits. About 3 days ago, his condition deteriorated, with inability of supine during nights, fever, cough, expectoration and a body temperature of 38.5 °C. By physical examination on admission, he was in a state of stupor, shortness of breath, heart rate 115/min, dullness by percussion of the right lung, coarse breathing sound of both lungs, dry rales of both lungs that predominantly right lung. Chest X-ray demonstrated multiple patches of opacity in both lungs that predominantly in the right lung. By laboratory tests, WBC 6.07×10^9/L, LY% 19.92 %, CK 1431U/L, LDH 988U/L, CRP 58.8 mg/L, $CD3^+$ $CD8^+$ 36.6 %, $CD3^-$ $CD56^+$ 15.9 %.

Within 2–5 days after onset, the condition deteriorated rapidly, with occurrence of severe pneumonia and multiple organs dysfunction. In addition to the laboratory finding of H7N9 nucleic acid positive, he was diagnosed with human infected H7N9 avian influenza. After therapies of anti-viral therapy, anti-inflammatory therapy, the use of hormones and mechanical ventilation as well as symptomatic therapies for multiple organs dysfunction, his condition was obviously improved. Ten days after his hospitalization, tracheal incubation was removed, consecutive nucleic acid tests for 3 times showed negative, and the indeces for routine blood test, heart function, liver function and kidney function were within normal limits. He was then discharge after hospitalization for 28 days. Six months later, he began to experience superior tracheal stenosis, which was treated by tracheal stent implantation.

[Imaging manifestations] Fig. 11.7

[Diagnosis] Pneumonia induced by human infected H7N9 avian influenza.

[Discussion]

The diagnostic evidence for this case is as the following:

1. The patient reported a history of contact to secretions and excretions of poultry. And his condition developed rapidly, with the occurrence of severe pneumonia, multiple organs dysfunction, persistent increase of the body temperature since d 5 after onset. By laboratory tests, he showed no increase of WBC count but decrease of lymphocyte count, and H7N9 nucleic acid positive.
2. By chest X-ray and CT scan, he showed multiple flakes of ground glass like and consolidation opacities in both lungs with air bronchogram. The lesions were in both lower lungs, predominantly the right lung, that progress rapidly and distribute extensively.
3. After 10 days treatment by anti-viral therapy, use of hormones and mechanical ventilation, the lung lesions were absorbed and improved. Consecutive nucleic acid test for H7N9 for 3 times showed negative.

Radiological evidence for the diagnosis is as the following:

1. The saliva acid of poultry, specifically binding to H7N9 avian influenza virus is mainly located in the lower respiratory tract, namely the lungs, but none in the upper respiratory tract. Human infection of H7N9 avian influenza virus directly induces pneumonia, with radiological signs of pneumonia early after onset.
2. Early after onset, the lesions may be confined within one lung, the most commonly the right lung. If both lungs involved, the lesions distribute in multiple segments and multiple lung lobes that are predominantly and more serious in the right lung. In addition, the lesions in both lower lungs are more serious than in both upper lungs, which is possibly related to the posture for radiology and the anatomy of trachea. Radiologically, both the parenchymal and interstitial lesions are demonstrated as large consolidation, interlobular septal thickening, and sporadic ground glass opacity, with air bronchogram.
3. During the progressive stage, human infected H7N9 avian influenza virus invades the lung tissues to induce the cytokine storm due to the absence of immunity to the new virus. Therefore, systematic inflammatory responses are triggered, with subsequent occurrence of acute respiratory distress syndrome (ARDS), shock and multiple organs failure. Radiologically, the lesions in lungs rapidly develop to involve multiple segments and lobes. Due to diffuse alveolar damages, chest X-ray and CT scan demonstrate extensively distributed ground glass opacity and consolidation opacity in both lungs, with air bronchogram, predominantly in both lower lungs or the right upper lung. In some cases, subpleural line and/or interlobular septal thickening is demonstrated; and in some other cases, pleural effusion. Pneumothorax and mediastinal lymphadenectasis may also be demonstrated.
4. During the convalescent stage, the lung lesions are demonstrated with slow absorption, shrinkage, and lightening in color after active anti-viral therapy and

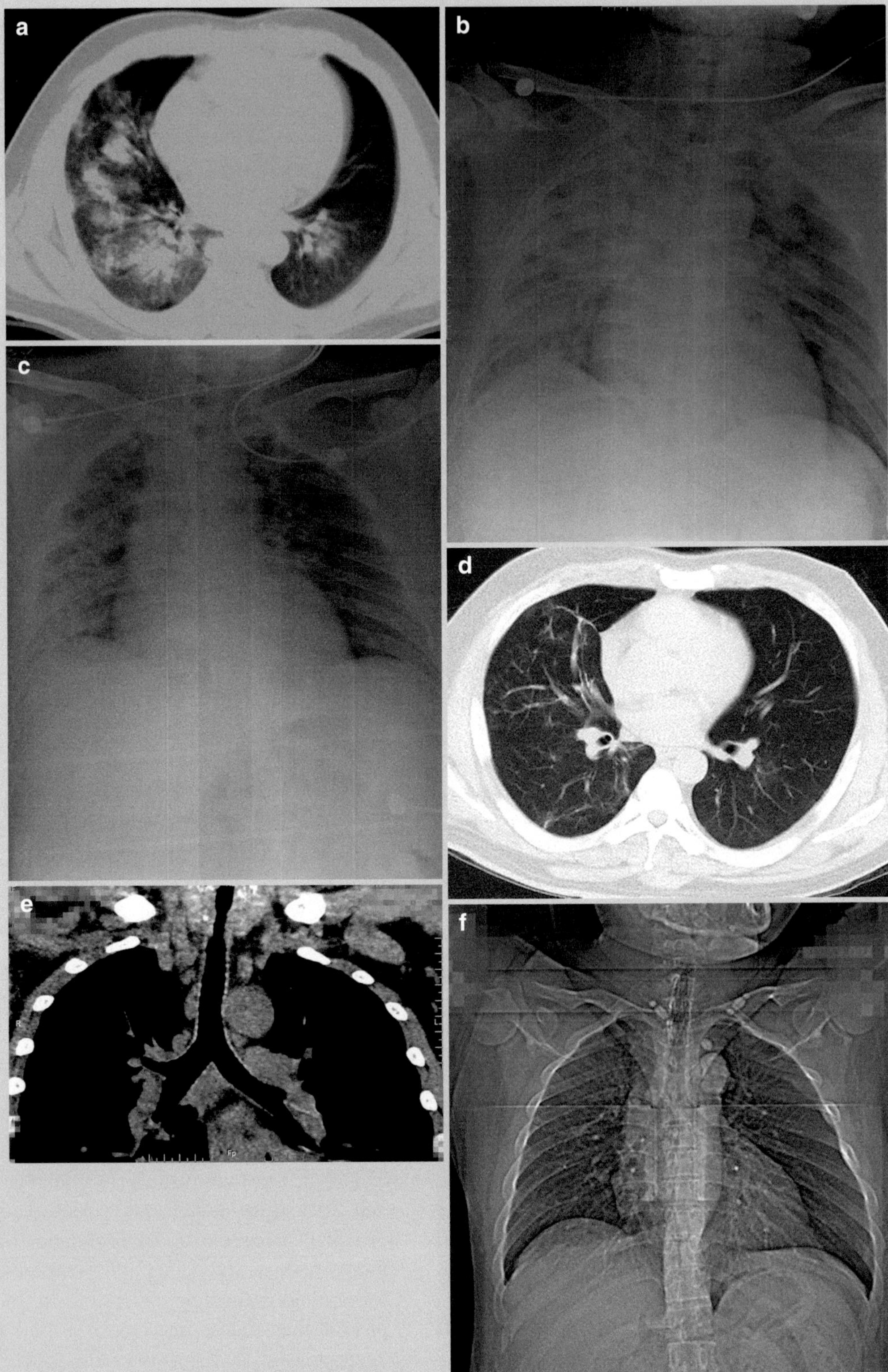

Fig. 11.7 On d 3 after onset, CT scan demonstrated nodular and flakes of consolidation opacity in the right lower lung, with air bronchogram inside; nodular consolidation in a small quantity in the left lower lung (**a**). On d 5 after onset, the lesions progressed rapidly. Chest X-ray showed multiple flakes of consolidation in both lungs that was predominantly in the right lung (**b**). On d 19 after onset, the respiratory symptoms were improved. Chest X-ray showed absorption and decrease of the consolidation (**c**). Reexamination 2 months after onset, the patient was cured and discharged. CT scan showed fibrous cords like opacity in a small quantity in both lower lungs (**d**). Reexamination 6 months after onset, the patient began to experience chest distress again. Coronary reconstruction following tracheal CT scan showed superior tracheal stenosis, possibly related to tracheal intubation (**e**). Chest distress was immediately alleviated after tracheal stent implantation (**f**)

respiratory supportive therapy, with increased transparency of the lungs. The flakes of and nodular parenchymal lesions are rapidly absorbed, while the grid like and cords like interstitial lesions are absorbed slowly. Pleural thickening may persist for a long period of time. Due to the chronic stimulation by tracheal incubation, the symptoms of tracheal stenosis may occur.

Human infected H7N9 avian influenza should be differentiated from the following diseases.

1. Type A H1N1 influenza
   Its early radiological signs include predominant GGO surrounding bronchovascular tree or in the subpleural area. And the lesions progress into extensive alveolar consolidation. Both pathologically and clinically, the changes are mild, with occurrence of death due to ARDS in rare critically ill patients. During the early stage of human infected H7N9 avian influenza, singular or multiple exudative lesions in multiple segments or lobes rapidly progress into ARDS and even multiple organs dysfunction. The diagnosis can be defined based on nucleic acid test of the virus.
2. Sever acute respiratory syndrome (SARS)
   Radiologically, both lungs are demonstrated with diffuse GGO and extensive consolidation. The lesions progress rapidly, mostly distribute in the lungs periphery and mainly involve the subpleural area. The interstitial lesions of SARS are more obvious than those of human infected H7N9 avian influenza, with interlobular septal thickening in paving-stones sign by HRCT.
3. Bacterial infection
   In the cases of lobar pneumonia, both WBC and neutrophil counts show significant increase. The lesions commonly involve one lung, more commonly the right lung, and multiple lobes involvement is rare. During its consolidation period, the lesions are commonly dense with air bronchogram. However, human infected H7N9 avian influenza is characterized by WBC count within normal limits and decreased lymphocyte count. The lesions rapidly develop into consolidations in multiple segments and lobes as well as ARDS. Thoracic bacterial infection may occur during treatment due to poor immunity of the patient, tracheal intubation and the use of hormones in a large quantity.

Case 8

[Brief Case History]

A 56-year-old man complained of fever (with the highest body temperature of 39.5 °C), sore throat and muscle soreness for 6 days with no known causes. His condition was hardly improved after anti-viral and symptomatic therapies, with occurrence of cough and expectoration for 2 days as well as chest distress, shortness of breath and consciousness disturbance for 1 day. Arterial blood gas analysis indicated respiratory acidosis and carbon dioxide retention. He reported no history of contact to poultry but a medical history of thymoma and its surgical removal.

[Radiological demonstration] Fig. 11.8

[Diagnosis] Pneumonia induced by human infected H7N9 avian influenza; severe pneumonia; type II respiration failure.

[Discussion]

After onset of clinical symptoms, the patient was diagnosed with ordinary influenza and corresponding therapy was given, with no obvious therapeutic efficacy. He paid no attention to his condition until its deterioration and received anti-viral therapy and respiratory supportive therapy. The initial radiological examination showed lobar and segmental consolidation of one lung, which resembles to those in the consolidation period of lobar pneumonia. After 6 days, the pulmonary lesions obviously progressed and were diffusely distributed in both lungs. In the following radiological examinations, the lesions deteriorated again, with gradual deterioration following slight absorption of the lesions and subsequent slow absorption. Based on clinical manifestations and laboratory tests, it was speculated that it may be related to occurrence of mixed infection in the late stage of the disease. Long-term following up observation indicated that the lesions are subject to interstitial fibrosis after their absorption.

In this case, differential diagnosis should be made from lobar pneumonia during its early stage. But it is challenging because both diseases show extremely similar radiological signs. However, in the patients with lobar pneumonia, clinical symptoms and signs can be obviously improved after administration of antibiotics and symptomatic therapy. But in this case, active therapies showed no obvious therapeutic efficacy, and the condition of the patient aggravated. Such outcomes should be paid focused attention and its etiological evidence should be traced to change therapeutic regime.

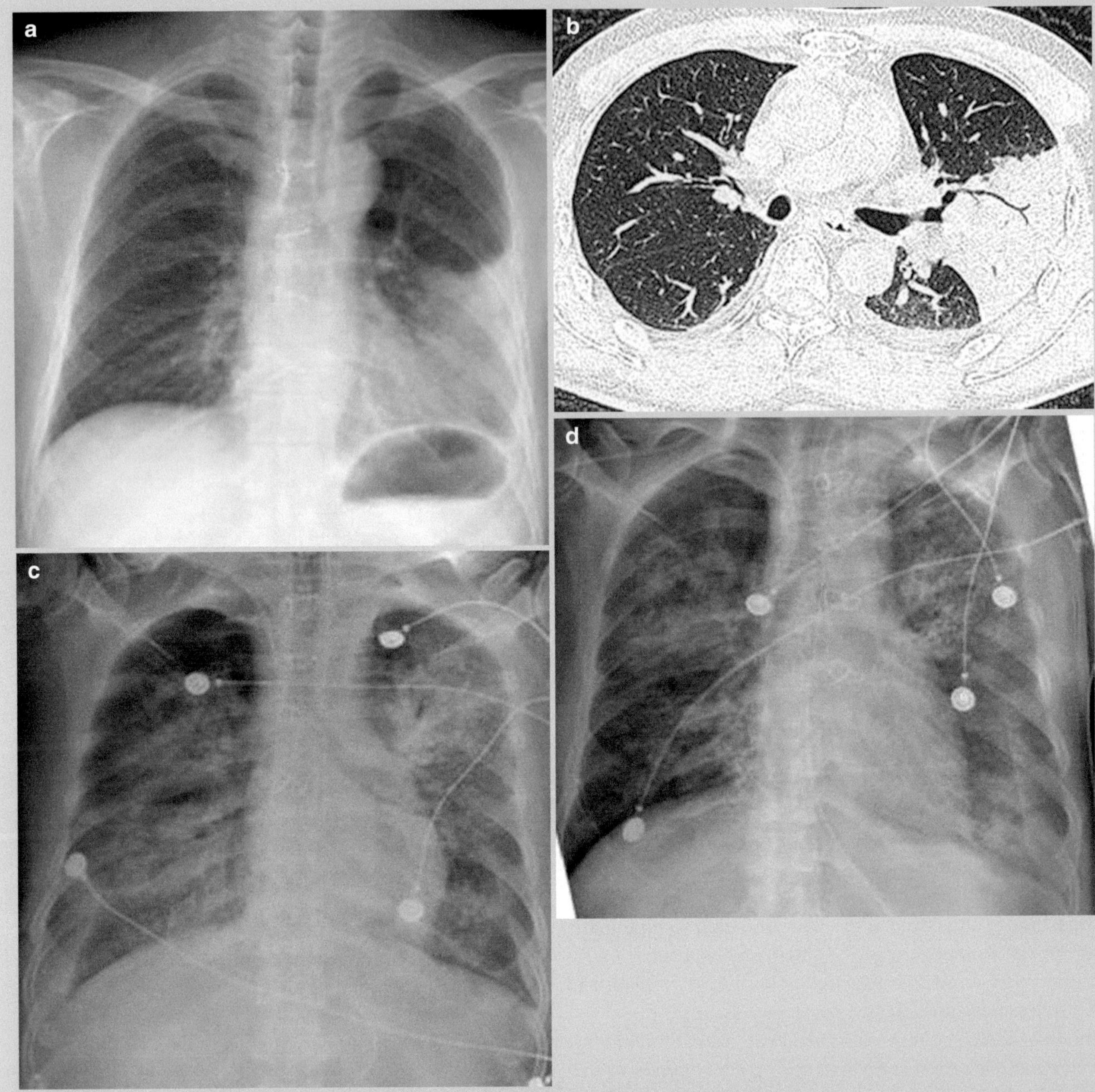

Fig. 11.8 On d 7 after onset, anterior-posterior chest X-ray demonstrated lobar segmental consolidation in the left lower lung field (**a**). CT scan showed consolidation in the left upper lung lobe, with air bronchogram inside (**b**). On d 13 after onset, bedside chest X-ray showed diffuse flakes of consolidation and ground glass opacity in both lungs (**c**). On d 18 after onset, bedside chest X-ray showed absorption of the lesions in the right lower lung but aggravating lesions in the left lower lung (**d**). On d 28 after onset, CT scan showed large consolidation in both lungs and aggravated consolidation in the right lower lung, with interlobular septal thickening (**e**). On d 31 after onset, bedside chest X-ray demonstrated absorption of the lesions in the left lung in grid like and honeycomb like changes (**f**). On d 32 after onset, CT scan showed interstitial thickening predominantly in the left upper lung, slightly decreased density of consolidation in the left lower lung, and obvious consolidation in the right lung (**g**). By reexamination 18 months after the onset, CT scan showed a small quantity of residual fibrous cords like opacity, indicating fibrosis (**h**)

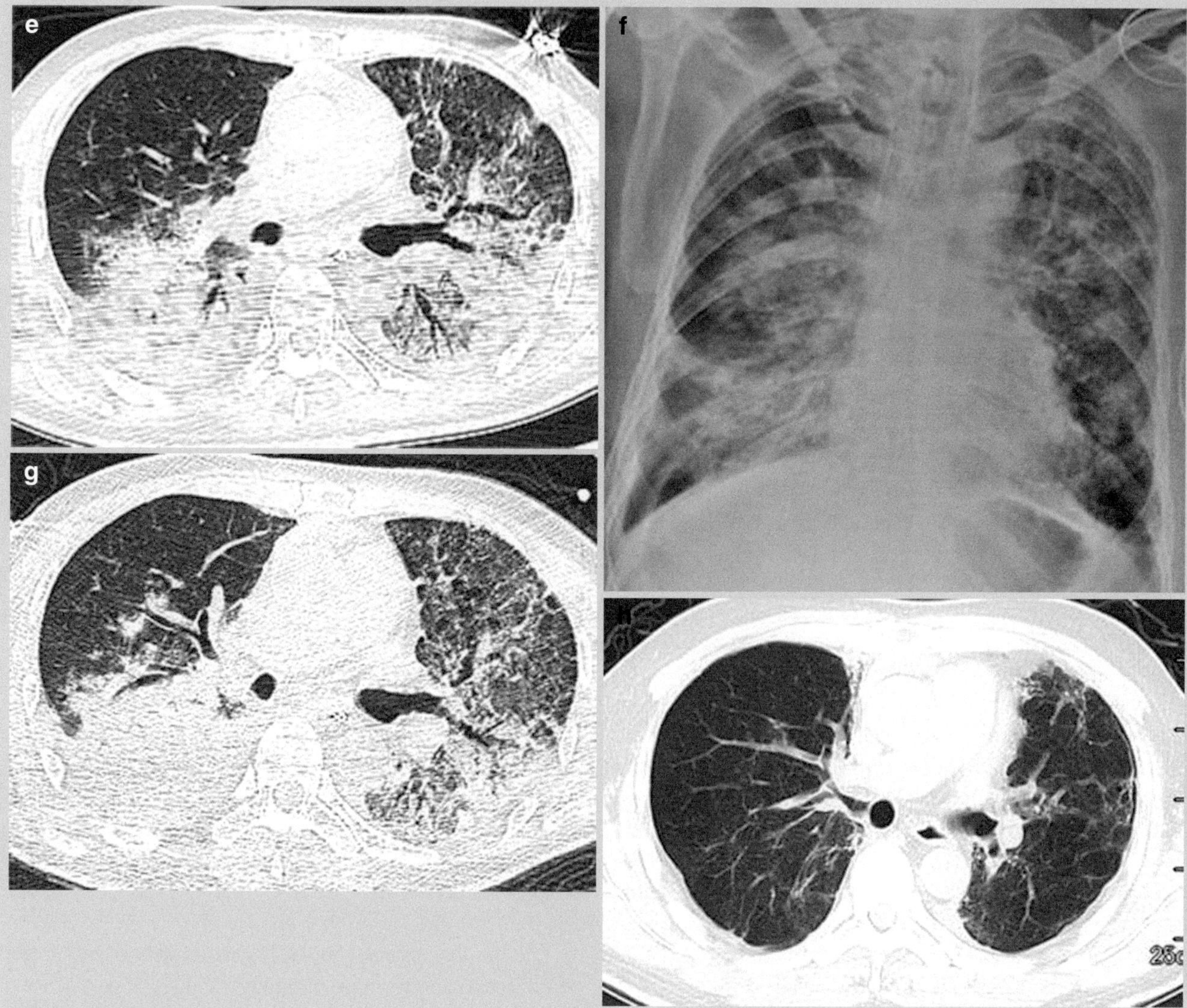

Fig. 11.8 (continued)

Case 9

[Brief Case History]

A 38-year-old man complained of fever with no known causes with the highest body temperature of 39.4 °C since Dec. 9, 2013, accompanying paroxysmal cough and expectoration of yellowish white thick sputum in a small quantity. He paid a clinic visit in a local hospital. But on Dec. 12, 2013, he was hospitalized due to aggravation of the condition. Chest X-ray showed large consolidation in the left lower lung and sporadic patches of opacity in the right lung. One day after treatment, these symptoms aggravated. Blood gas analysis showed type I respiratory failure. After that, the patient was transferred into ICU. By physical examination on admission, his body temperature 36.1 °C, heart rate 116/min, breathing rate 36/min, and blood pressure 116/67 mmHg. He respirated with the assistance of ventilators and showed no response to calling. Conjunctiva slightly swollen in both eyes, with no congestion, no yellowish sclera, equal size of bilateral pupils in a diameter of about 2 mm that are sensitive to light. Pharynx congested, bilateral tonsils no swelling, no special abnormality in heart examination. Fremitus weakened at the left chest, no sensation of pleural friction; dullness of the left lower lung by percussion; coarse breathing sounds of both lungs that was relatively weaker in the left lung; fine moist rales in both lungs. He reported a history of buying chicken in a market and cooking it on Nov. 20, 2013. Routine blood test showed WBC 3.48×10^9/L, GR% 76.1 %. Blood biochemistry revealed CK 3319U/L, LDH 882U/L, CKMB 32.5U/L, K^+ 2.83 mmol/L, Na^+ 133 nmol/L, troponin and BNP within normal limits, CRP 26.71 mg/L, ALT 136U/L, AST 470U/L, ALB 27 g/L. Blood gas analysis showed pH 7.48, PO_2 47 mmHg, PCO_2 25.4 mmHg, and BE -5 mmol/L. CD4 T cell count was 42/μl. By etiological examination, his tracheal aspirates showed H7N9 nucleic acid positive.

[Radiological demonstration] Fig. 11.9

[Diagnosis] Pneumonia induced by human infected H7N9 avian influenza.

[Discussion]

For this case, the symptoms and signs are in line with the diagnostic criteria of severe pneumonia induced by human infected H7N9 avian influenza established by the National Health and Family Planning Commission of China. At the early stage, the patient showed pulmonary consolidation, with complication of pleural effusion. And radiologically, the lesions are characterized by the following:

1. On d 3 after onset, plain chest X-ray showed poorly defined patches of opacity in the left middle and lower lung fields as well as left pleural effusion; ground glass opacity in the right middle lung field. Chest CT scan on the same day demonstrated patches of ground glass opacity in the right middle lung lobe and the left upper lung; large consolidation in the left lower lung lobe, with air bronchogram inside.
2. On d 14 after onset, the lesion of lung consolidation was obviously absorbed, with patches of GGO in the right upper and middle lung and the left upper lung, predominantly in the subpleural areas; the lesion of consolidation in the left lower lung was absorbed compared to previous CT scan findings. And the air opacity in the anterior mediastinum and the anterior thoracic wall is induced by invasive ventilation.
3. Reexamination by chest CT scan on d 39 after onset revealed almost absorbed GGO in both lungs and consolidation in the left lower lung; but observable lesions of pulmonary interstitial fibrosis, such as small GGO in lower lungs and interlobular septal thickening. In addition, the gas opacity in the anterior mediastinum and anterior thoracic wall was also absorbed.

Pneumonia induced by H7N9 avian influenza should be differentiated from other emerging infectious diseases, such as viral pneumonia induced by H5N1 avian influenza virus and type A H1N1 influenza virus as well as SARS. Radiologically, they share commonalities of GGO and consolidation, with rapid change and progression. Early lesions of pneumonia induced by H7N9 avian influenza are predominantly located in both lower lungs, which is not characteristic of pneumonia induced by H5N1 avian influenza virus or type A H1N1 influenza virus and SARS. Therefore, its differential diagnosis based on radiology is challenging, and clinical diagnosis should be defined based on epidemiological investigation and etiological examination.

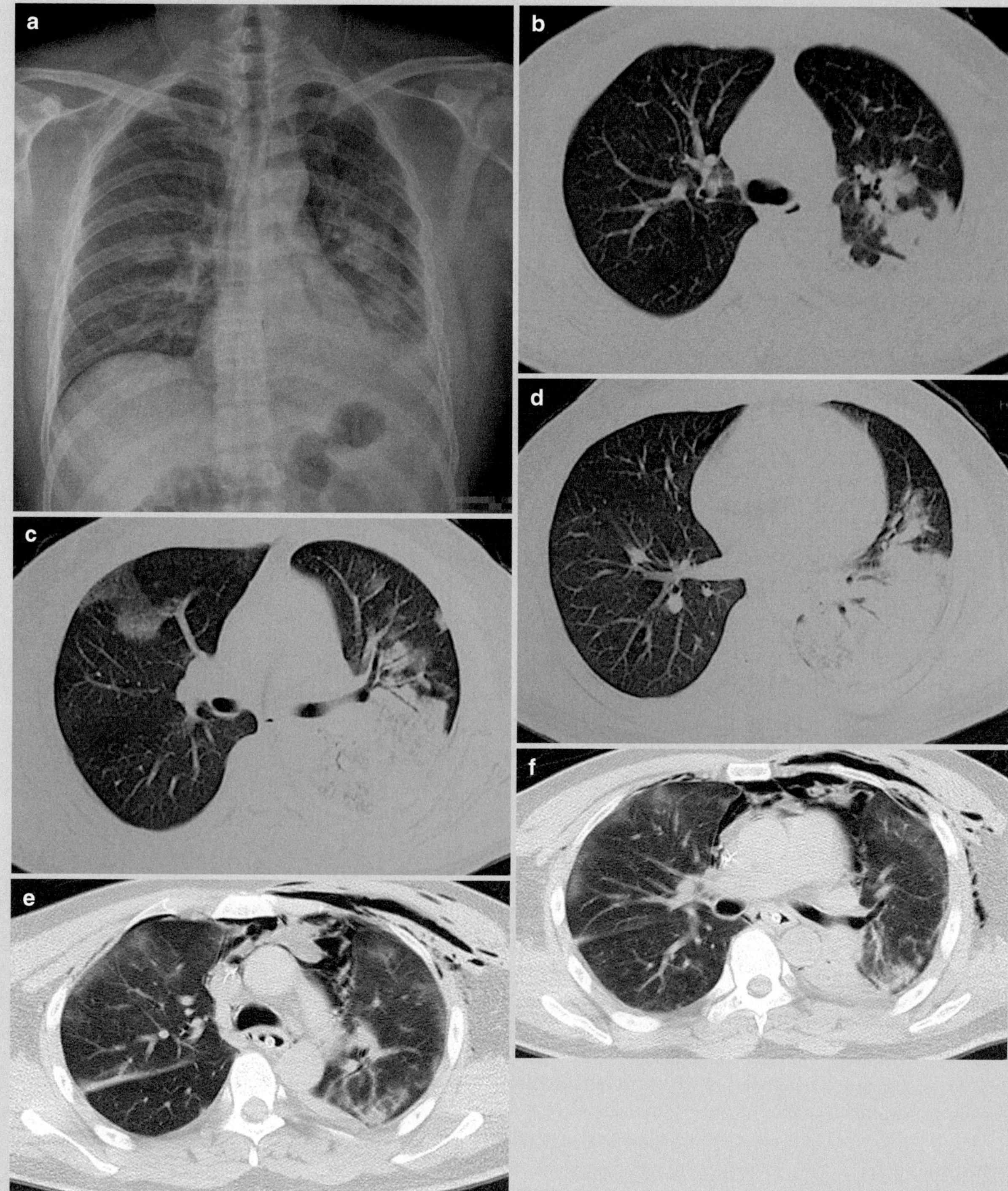

Fig. 11.9 On d 3 after onset, chest X-ray showed large flakes of high density opacity in the left middle and lower lung fields, with poorly defined boundary; flakes of ground glass opacity in the right middle lung field; and blunt left costophrenic angle (**a**). On d 3, chest CT scan showed irregular flakes of opacity in the apical posterior segment of left upper lung lobe (**b**). Patches of ground glass opacity in the right middle lung lobe and the left upper lung lobe; large consolidation in the left lower lung lobe (**c**). Shrinkage of the left lower lung lobe was shown, with large consolidation and air bronchogram inside (**d**). On d 14, chest CT scan demonstrated flakes of ground glass opacity in both upper lungs; gas opacity in the anterior mediastinum and the thoracic wall (**e**). Ground glass opacity was observable under the pleura in the right middle lung lobe and the left upper lung; flakes of consolidation adjacent to the chest aorta in the left lower lung lobe; gas opacity in the anterior mediastinum and the thoracic wall (**f**). Pleural effusion in a small quantity was detected in the right pleural cavity; large consolidation in the left lower lung with air bronchogram inside; gas opacity in the anterior mediastinum and the left anterior thoracic wall (**g**). On d 39, chest CT scan demonstrated interlobular septal thickening in the dorsal segment of the left lower lung lobe, with local pleural thickening (**h**). Flakes of ground glass opacity was observed in the dorsal segment of left lower lung lobe, predominantly in the left lower lung lobe (**i**)

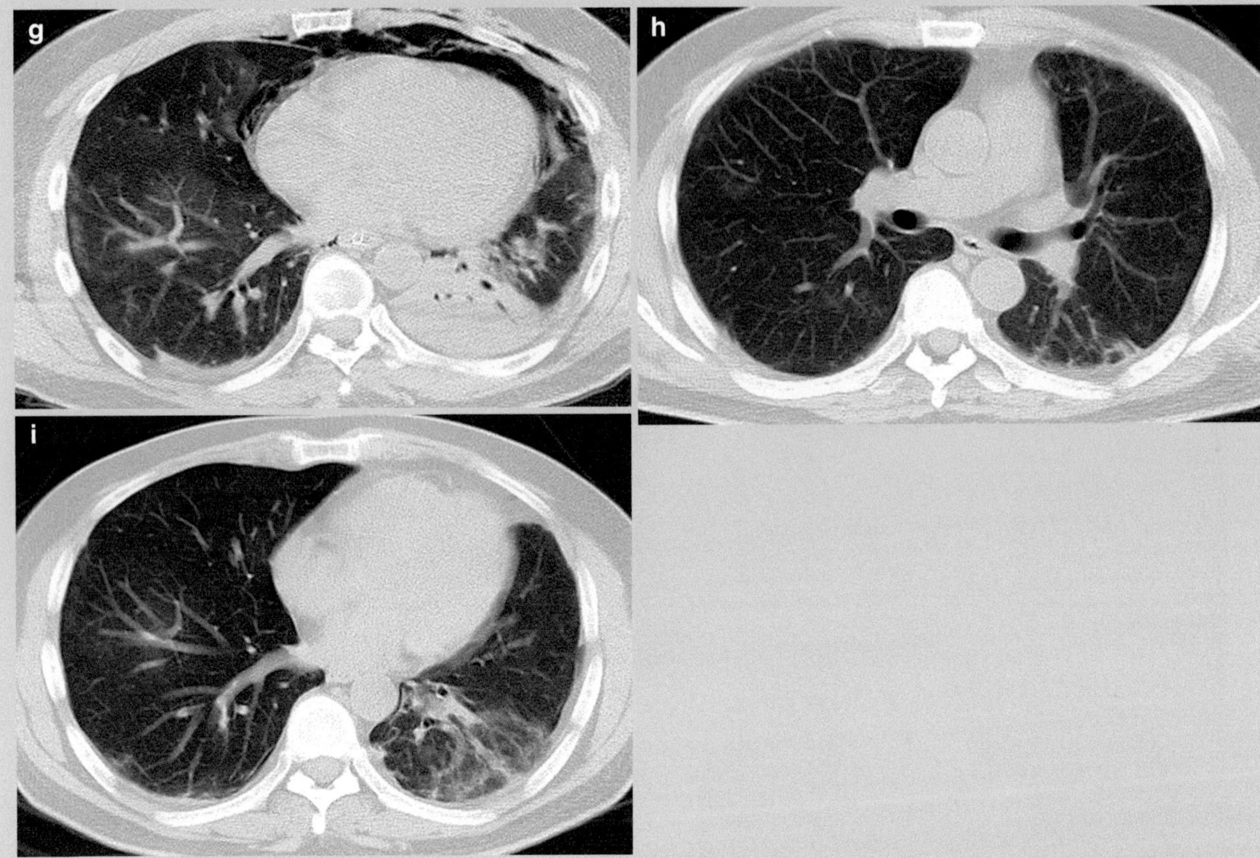

Fig. 11.9 (continued)

Case 10

[Brief Case History]

A 55-year-old man experienced frequent paroxysmal cough and expectoration of a little yellowish white thick sputum since Jan. 5, 2014. His condition was diagnosed as hypertension due to a blood pressure of 154/96 mmHg and he received medication to lower his blood pressure. Several days later, he was hospitalized on Jan. 10, 2014 due to the aggravating condition. Chest X-ray revealed bronchiectasis in the left lower lung with accompanying infection, which was then considered as lung infection. He was then admitted to the Respiratory Department for treatment, but his cough was not improved by anti-infection therapy. On Jan. 13, 2014, he still experienced fever, with the highest body temperature of 38 °C. An immediate blood gas analysis indicated respiratory failure, and he was transferred to ICU for tracheal intubation and assisted breathing via ventilator. Bedside chest X-ray revealed extensive infection in both lungs and possible bronchiectasis in left lower lung, indicating significant progression compared to the condition on Jan. 10, 2014. Routine blood test showed WBC count 2.61×10^9/L, GR% 70.9 %, RBC count 5.0×10^{12}/L, HGB 158 g/L, PLT 71×10^9/L. Blood gas analysis revealed pH 7.45, PO_2 50 mmHg, and PCO_2 24 mmHg. On Jan. 13, 2014, laboratory test by CDC showed reported alveolar lavage fluid positive to H7N9 avian influenza virus, and peripheral CD4 T cell count 66/μl.

[Radiological demonstration] Fig. 11.10

[Diagnosis] Pneumonia induced by human infected H7N9 avian influenza.

[Discussion]

In this case, the patient was an elderly man with no definitive history of contact to live poultry. The onset symptoms include cough and expectoration, and laboratory tests showed decreased peripheral WBC count, decreased platelet count, and decreased blood potassium level. On d 5 after onset, chest X-ray revealed infection in the left lower lung. The patient experienced repeated fever and the condition rapidly progressed into respiratory failure, multiple organs failure and infectious shock.

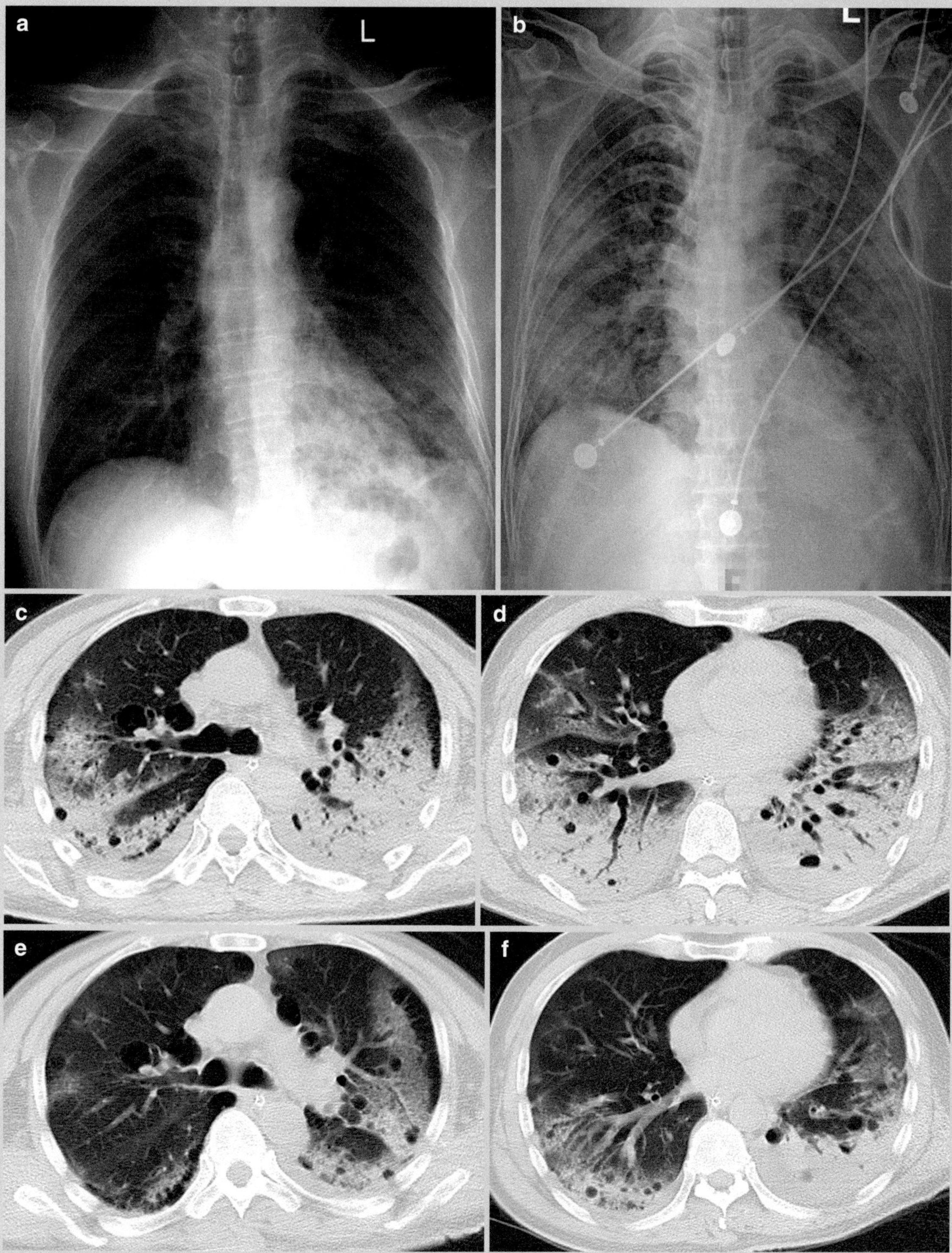

Fig. 11.10 On d 5 after onset, chest X-ray showed poorly defined patches of high density opacity in the left lower lung field; overlapping of some lesions with heart shadow (**a**). On d 8 after onset, chest X-ray showed flakes of ground glass opacity in both lungs, and consolidation in the bilateral middle and lower lung fields (**b**). On d 9 after onset, chest CT scan showed multiple large high density opacity and ground glass opacity in both lower lung lobes, predominantly in the left lower lung lobe (**c**). Large consolidation was revealed in both lower lungs, with air bronchogram and multiple cystic translucent areas (**d**). On d 14, chest CT scan showed unevenly distributed ground glass opacity in the bilateral upper and middle lung lobes, consolidation in the left upper lung with multiple small translucent areas with no wall (**e**). Both lower lungs were revealed with patches of GGO like high density opacity and the left lower lung was shown with large consolidation and round translucent opacity in different sizes inside. They were mainly distributed in the left subpleural area and the dorsal lungs. Compared to the chest CT scan film 5 days ago, the lesions were absorbed (**f**). On d 209, the left lung was shown with unevenly distributed ground glass opacity; the left subpleural area and anterior mediastinum were shown with lung bullae (**h**). Lung bullae were sporadic in both lower lung lobes (**h**)

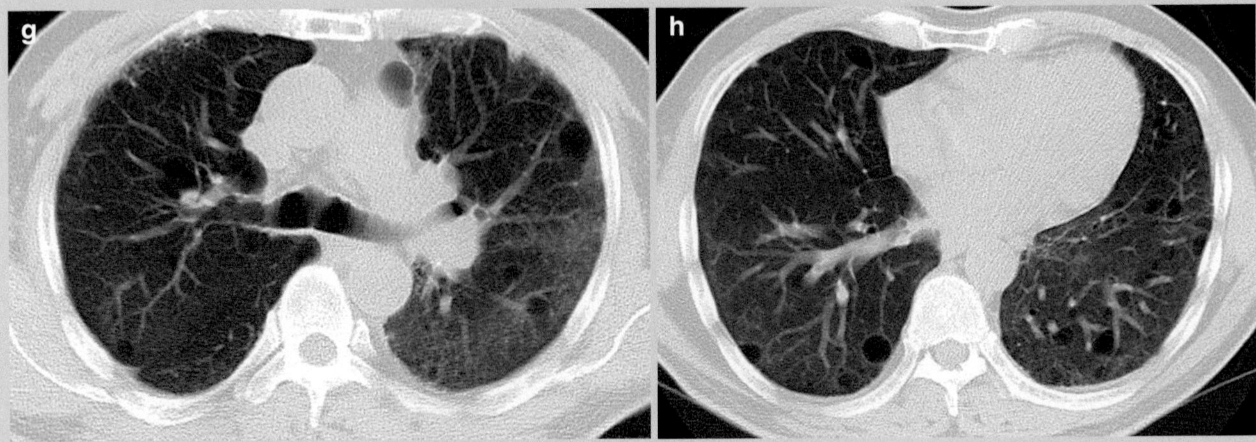

Fig. 11.10 (continued)

On d 5 after onset, chest X-ray indicated infection in the left lower lung and on d 8 after onset, the lesions spread to involve both lungs. On d 9 after onset, chest CT scan revealed large consolidation and ground glass opacity in each lobe of both lungs, with multiple small translucent areas inside. These radiological signs indicated rapid progression of the lesions, which are rarely observed in patients with bacterial and common viral pneumonia.

This case is radiologically characterized by the followings:

1. The lung lesions are mainly consolidation and GGO, which emerge early after onset. And the lesions are mainly distributed in the subpleural area of both lower lung lobes. Air bronchogram is observable in the consolidation opacity.
2. The lesions progress rapidly but are absorbed slowly. The lesions are firstly confined within one lung, but rapidly spread to involve lobes and segments of both lungs. The condition rapidly develops into respiratory failure. With the use of various therapies, the lung lesions are gradually absorbed, with slower absorption of interstitial lesions than parenchymal lesions.

Case 11

[Brief Case History]

A 39-year-old woman experienced cough and expectoration of yellowish sputum with no known causes since Jan. 15, 2014. Her condition was not improved after treatment in a local hospital on Jan. 17. And she was then hospitalized in a superior hospital due to a diagnosis of lung infection. Physical examinations showed a body temperature of 38 °C, heart rate 95/min, respiration rate 19/min and blood pressure 123/73 mmHg. She was well conscious in good spirits, no shortness of breath, and cooperative to the physical examinations. By palpation, the swallow lymph nodes no enlarged, and 3 depression sign negative (−). Pharynx congested, bilateral tonsils no swollen with no pus spots, and oral cavity no Koplik's spot. The chest no malformation, bilateral breathing mobility equal, breathing sounds of both lung coarse, moist rales in the right lower lung, and no pleural friction sounds. The heart beat rhythm regular, and no murmurs by auscultation. The abdomen was soft, liver and spleen unpalpable under ribs, the whole abdomen no tenderness and rebound, and bowel sound normal. Both lower limbs no swollen. She denied medical histories of other diseases but experienced vomiting, nausea and pruritus of right lower leg after oral intake of Cephaloridine 1 day ago. She also denied a history of contact to live poultry, but reported a history of eating chickens 6 days ago. Routine blood test showed WBC count 5.2×10^9/L, GR% 63 %, and LY% 30.1 %. Blood gas analysis revealed pH 7.47, PCO_2 31 mmHg, PO_2 67 mmHg, Na^+ 134 mmol/L, K^+ 2.7 mmol/L, and Ca^{2+} 0.91 mmol/L. Sputum test showed nucleic acid of H7N9 avian influenza virus positive.

[Radiological demonstration] Fig. 11.11

[Diagnosis] Pneumonia induced by H7N9 avian influenza.

[Discussion]

This case is radiologically characterized by the followings:

1. On d 2 after onset, chest plain X-ray showed small flake of high density opacity at the cardiodiaphragmatic angle of right lower lung field, indicating emergence of lesions in lower lung in the early stage of pneumonia induced by human infected H7N9 avian influenza. On d 3 after onset, chest X-ray further proved flake of GGO in the posterior basilar segment of right lower lung lobe, and opacity with mixed GGO density with parenchymal density.
2. On d 6 after onset, chest CT scan demonstrated rapid progression of the lesions in both lungs, with large consolidation in the right lower lung lobe and sporadic poorly defined patches of opacity in the right middle lung lobe and each basilar segment of the left lower lung lobe. Within 72 h, the progression of lesions was more than 50 %, which was in line with the diagnostic criteria of severe pneumonia induced by human infected H7N9 avian influenza.
3. At the peak of lesion progression, the lesions began to be absorbed after effective therapy was given, but the convalescent stage lasted for a relatively long period of time. On d 31 after onset, chest CT scan showed absorption of most lesions but still residual cords like opacity and small GGO in the subpleural area of posterior basilar segment in the right lower lung lobe.

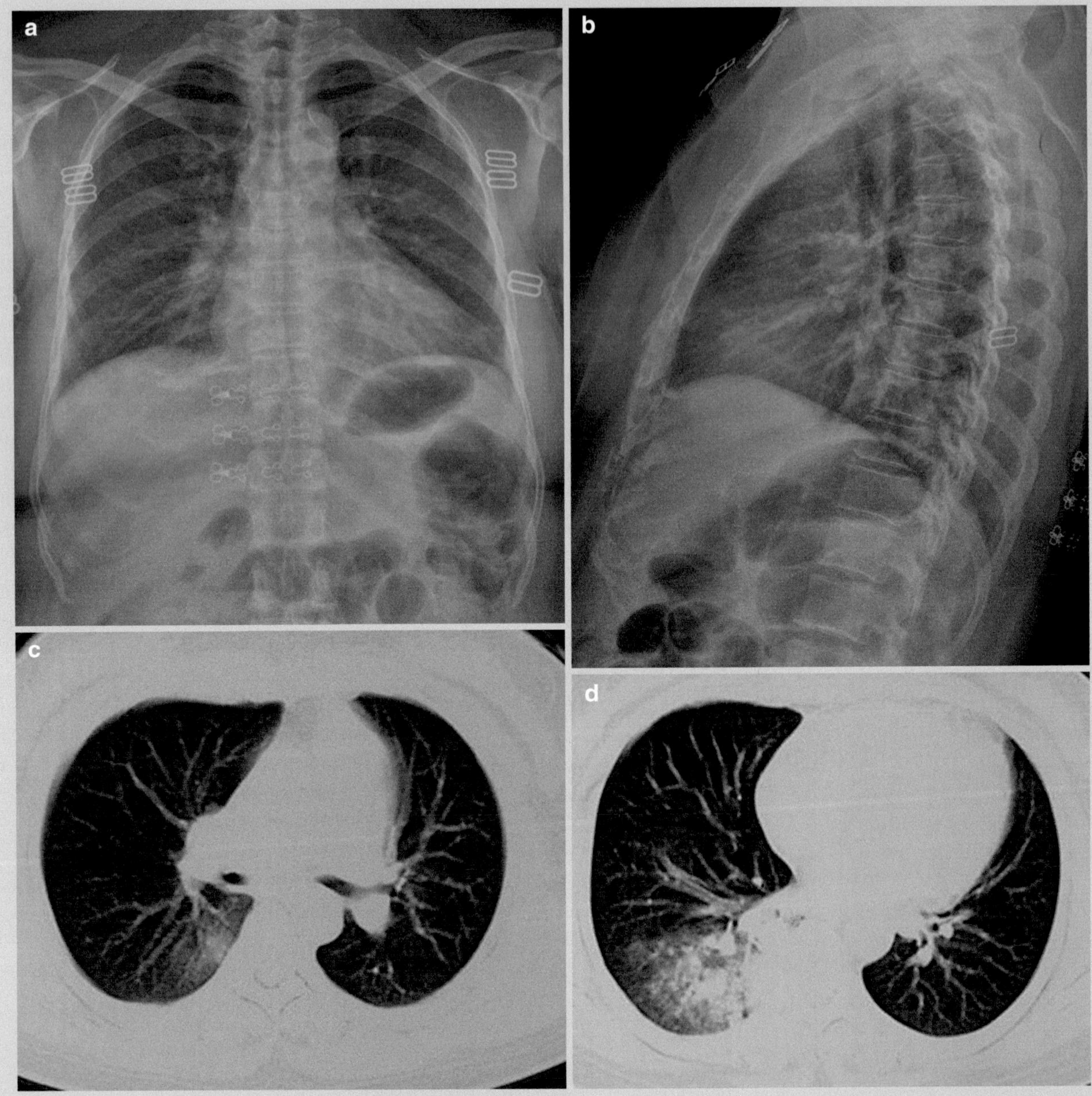

Fig. 11.11 On d 2 after onset, anterior-posterior and lateral X-ray showed poorly defined small flake of high density opacity near the cardiodiaphragmatic angle in the right lower lung field. And lateral X-ray demonstrated poorly defined small flake of opacity in the overlapping area of posterior costophrenic angle and thoracic vertebrae in the right lower lung field (**a**, **b**). On d 3 after onset, chest CT scan showed flake of ground glass opacity in the posterior basilar segment of right lower lung lobe (**c**). The right lower lung lobe was revealed with large flake of opacity with mixed GGO density and parenchymal density (**d**). On d 6 after onset, chest CT scan demonstrated large consolidation in the posterior basilar segment of right lower lung (**e**). The right middle and lower lung was revealed with large consolidation with air bronchogram inside. The left lower lung was revealed with flake of consolidation and ground glass like high density opacity. Compared to the chest CT scan film 3 days ago, the lesions significantly progressed (**f**). On d 31 after onset, chest CT scan demonstrated absorbed consolidation opacity in the right lower lung lobe at the bronchial bifurcating level (**g**). The right lower lung lobe was revealed with GGO like opacity and interstitial fibrous cords like opacity near diaphragmatic dome. The left lingual lung lobe was revealed with GGO like opacity and interstitial fibrous cords like opacity (**h**)

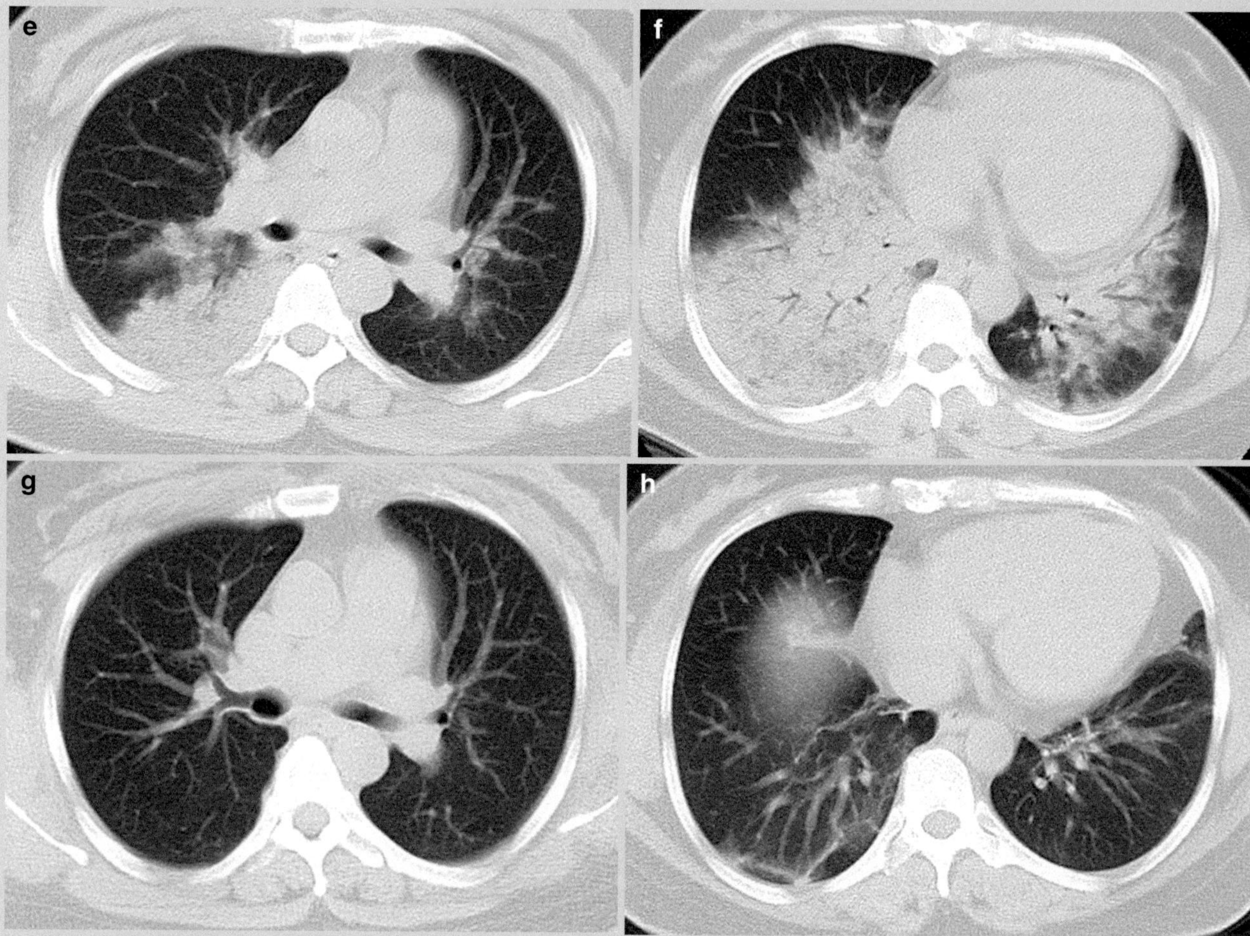

Fig. 11.11 (continued)

References

Ajlan AM, Quiney B, Nicolaou S, et al. Swine-origin influenza A(H1N1)viral infection: radiographic and CT findings. AJR Am J Roentgenol. 2009;193(6):1494–9.

Cai RP, Du RB, Li T. Radiological demonstrations of lung lesions and their dynamic changes in human infected H7N9 avian influenza. J Trauma Emerg (Electronic Version). 2014;2(3):19–22.

Chen Y, Liang W, Yang S, et al. Human infections with the emerging avian influenza A H7N9 virus from wet market poultry: clinical analysis and characterisation of viral genome. Lancet. 2013;381(9881):1916–25.

Feng F, Jiang Y, Yuan M, et al. Association of radiologic findings with mortality in patients with avian influenza H7N9 pneumonia. PLoS One. 2013;9(4), e93885.

Gao R, Cao B, Hu Y, et al. Human infection with a novel avian-origin influenza (H7N9) virus. N Engl J Med. 2013;368(24):1888–97.

Huang XR, Huang H, Lu PX, et al. CT scan demonstrations and their relationship with virus load and CD4 T cell count in pneumonia induced by human infected H7N9 avian influenza. J Radiol Pract. 2014a;29(7):751–5.

Huang XR, Zeng Z, Lu PX, et al. Radiological data analysis of pneumonia induced by human infected H7N9 avian influenza: report of 12 cases. J CT MRI China. 2014b;12(2):8–11.

Li HJ. Recent understandings and insights about the emerging infectious disease: human infected H7N9 avian influenza. Radiol Pract. 2014;29(7):738–9.

Li YF, Li HJ. Chest radiological demonstrations of human infected H7N9 avian influenza. Radiol Pract. 2014;29(7):745–7.

Li L, Li HJ, Zhao J, et al. Chest radiological data of human infected H7N9 avian influenza: report of 13 cases. Radiol Pract. 2014;29(7):748–50.

Lu PX, Zhou BP. Imaging diagnosis of emerging infectious diseases. Beijing: People's Medical Publishing House; 2013.

Lu PX, Zeng Z, Zheng FQ, et al. Radiological demonstrations of severe pneumonia induced by human infected H7N9 avian influenza and their dynamic changes. Radiol Pract. 2014;29(7): 740–4.

National Health and Family Planning Commission of P.R.China. Clinical Guideline for human infected H7N9 avian influenza (2014). Chin J Clin Infect Dis. 2014;7(1):1–3.

Song FX, Zhou J, Shi YX, et al. Bedside chest radiography of novel influenza A (H7N9) virus infections and follow-up findings after short-time treatment. Chin Med J (Engl). 2013;126(23): 4440–3.

Wang Q, Zhang Z, Shi Y, Jiang Y, et al. Emerging H7N9 influenza A (novel reassortant avian origin) pneumonia: radiologic findings. Radiology. 2013a;268(9):882–9.

Wang Y, Zhou ZP, Zhang YW, et al. Clinical and radiological features of human infected H7N9 avian influenza. Chin J Radiol. 2013b;47(9):780–2.

Wang YQ, Shi YX, Zhang ZY, et al. Primary radiological data analysis about pneumonia induced by human infected H7N9 avian influenza. Chin J Radiol. 2013c;47(6):505–8.

Wang XM, Hu S, Hu CH, et al. Chest imaging of H7N9 subtype of human avian influenza. Radiol Infect Dis. 2015;1(2):51–6.

Xin XY, Chang Y, Sun XM, et al. Chest radiological demonstrations of pneumonia induced by H7N9 avian influenza virus. J Med Radiol. 2015;47(9):637–40.

Zeng Z, Lu PX, Zhou BP, et al. Radiological demonstrations of severe pneumonia induced by H7N9 avian influenza virus. J Tubelcu Lung Health. 2014;3(1):25–8.

Zhou BP, Li YM, Lu PX. Human infected avian influenza. Beijing: Science Press; 2007.

Human Infected H5N6 Avian Influenza

12

Puxuan Lu, Qingsi Zeng, Yue Zeng, and Qi An

12.1 Introduction

Human infected H5N6 avian influenza is an acute respiratory infectious disease caused by H5N6 subtype of avian influenza virus.

On May 6, 2014, throat swab of 1 patient with severe pneumonia showed positive to nucleic acid of H5N6 avian influenza virus in Nanchong, Sichuan, China. Further examination and test by CDC of China proved that the virus is H5N6 subtype of avian influenza virus. The patient reported a history of contact to dead poultry and was clinically diagnosed with acute severe pneumonia. And after emergency rescuing procedures, death still occurred in this patient and this is the first case of human infected H5N6 avian influenza worldwide.

On Dec. 23, 2014, the second case of human infected H5N6 avian influenza worldwide, also the first case in Guangdong province of China, was reported by the Provincial Health and Family Planning Commission in Guangdong. The patient, a 58-year-old man, bought a living chicken in a market and got caught in the rain all the way home on Dec. 22, 2014, and then the symptoms occurred. On the same day, further examination and test by CDC of China proved nucleic acid of H5N6 avian influenza virus positive. On the following day, consultation and analysis by experts group organized by the National Health and Family Planning Commission of China, in combination to the clinical manifestations, laboratory tests and epidemiological history, the diagnosis was defined to be human infected H5N6 avian influenza. After active therapies in designated hospital of Guangzhou for more than 1 month, the patient was exempted from quarantine and expected to be discharged in recent days.

The symptoms of human infected H5N6 avian influenza resemble to human infected H5N1 and H7N9 avian influenza. After onset, the condition rapidly develops into severe pneumonia, with early respiratory symptoms of fever (with a body temperature of above 38 °C) and cough. In the following 5–7 days after onset, severe pneumonia occurs, with symptoms like dyspnea, which progressively aggravates. Anti-viral medications, such as oseltamivir, are effective for human infected H5N6 avian influenza.

The subtype H5N6 of avian influenza virus is categorized into the family of Orthomyxoviridae and is segmental negative-stranded RNA virus. Other subtypes of avian influenza virus include H5N1 and H7N9 avian influenza viruses. On Aug. 28, 2014, gooses in the district of Shuangcheng (in Harbin, Heilongjiang province of China) showed symptoms like avian influenza, with 20550 sick gooses including 17790 deaths. By tests in the National Reference Laboratory of Avian Influenza, the disease was defined as highly pathogenic H5N6 avian influenza. By Dec. 31, 2014, 25 outbreaks of H5N6 avian influenza occurred in poultries nationwide, including Heilongjiang, Zhejiang, Hubei, Guangxi, Anhui, Guizhou, Tibet, Guangdong, Hunan, Hebei, Fujian and Yunnan provinces and Chongqing city. Some of the tested samples were from farms, and some from living poultries markets or their environment.

P. Lu (✉) • Q. An
Affiliated Shenzhen Third People's Hospital, Guangdong Medical College, Shenzhen, Guangdong, China
e-mail: lupuxuan@126.com

Q. Zeng
Affiliated First Hospital, Guangzhou Medical University, Guangzhou, Guangdong, China

Y. Zeng
Affiliated Hospital, Chuanbei Medical College, Nanchong, Sichuan, China

H. Li (ed.), *Radiology of Influenza*, DOI 10.1007/978-94-024-0908-6_12

12.2 Typical Cases

Case 1

[Brief Case History]
A 50-year-old man was hospitalized on Apr. 21, 2014 due to chief complaints of fever and cough for 8 days, dyspnea and bloody sputum for 1 day. At d 8 prior to his hospitalization (Apr. 13, 2014), he began to experience aversion to cold, fever (body temperature not reported), systemic soreness and runny nose. He then paid a visit in a local clinic and received oral intake of Chinese patent medicine for cold. However, his condition showed no obvious improvement. On Apr. 18, 2014, his symptoms obviously aggravated, with cough, aversion to cold, fever, systemic soreness, headache and accompanying poor appetite and malaise. After treatment by Compound Amionpyrine Antipyrine Injection and dexamethasone, his condition still showed no improvement. On Apr. 19, 2014, he began to experience abdominal upset, dyspnea, shortness of breath after physical activities, and expectoration of a little bloody sputum. On the following day, chest X-ray showed large consolidation in the left lung and nodular patches of opacity in the right upper lung. By the test of CDC in Nanyun, Sichuan province on Apr. 21, 2014, the nucleic acid of H5N6 avian influenza was shown positive. And death finally occurred on Apr. 22, 2014 after emergency rescuing procedures. By physical examination on admission, the body temperature was 37.3 °C, heart rate 96/min, breathing rate 30/min and blood pressure 106/74 mmHg. He showed complexion of acute disease, good consciousness, and poor spirits. By percussion, dull sound of the left lung and a little sporadic fine moist rales; while clear breathing sound of the right lung and no dry or moist rales. No other positive signs found. The patient was a farmer who had raised and saled poultries (including chickens and ducks) for a long time. He reported recent deaths of his poultries and a history of cooking and eating them. By routine blood test, WBC count 1.48×10^9/L, GR% 82.4%, and LY% 12.8%. By arterial blood glass analysis, PO_2 55.0 mmHg, PCO_2 34.0 mmHg, SaO_2 91.0%; CRP 252.00 mg/L, PCT 3.600 ng/ml. By blood biochemistry, AST 84.4U/L, and Cr 70.8 μmol/L. On May 6, 2014, the tests by the National CDC of China further proved the diagnosis of human infected H5N6 avian influenza.

[Radiological demonstration] Fig. 12.1

[Diagnosis] Pneumonia induced by human infected H5N6 avian influenza

[Discussion]
In this case, the patient was the first case of human infected H5N6 avian influenza worldwide, with acute onset and rapid progression. His clinical manifestations were characterized by:

1. Definitive epidemiological history of contact.
   The patient was a farmer who had raised and saled poultries (including chickens and ducks) for a long time. He reported recent deaths of poultries and a history of cooking and eating them.
2. He experienced influenza like symptoms, including fever, cough, dyspnea and accompanying expectoration of bloody sputum.
3. Acute onset and rapid progression.
   On d 7 after onset, the patient began to experience dyspnea and other symptoms of severe pneumonia, which progressively aggravated and finally developed into ARDS and death.

The radiological demonstrations are characterized by:

1. On d 8 after onset, chest CT scan showed that the lung lesions predominantly as consolidation and GGO, with multiple lobes and segments involved; obvious lesions in the lateral part of cortex.
2. On d 9 after onset, bedside chest X-ray demonstrated progression of lesions in the right lung, with enlarged areas of consolidation and GGO as well as lesions of ARDS. Meanwhile, pleural effusion in a small quantity in the left pleural cavity indicated progression of the disease.

Rapid progression and extensive lesions are the commonalities of pneumonia induced by type A influenza virus. In this first case of pneumonia induced by H5N6 avian influenza virus worldwide, due to our limited knowledge about radiological signs of the disease, its differential diagnosis from pneumonia induced by H7N9, H5N1, H5N6 avian influenza viruses and other type A influenza viruses is challenging. And the diagnosis was defined based mainly on the epidemiological history and etiological examination.

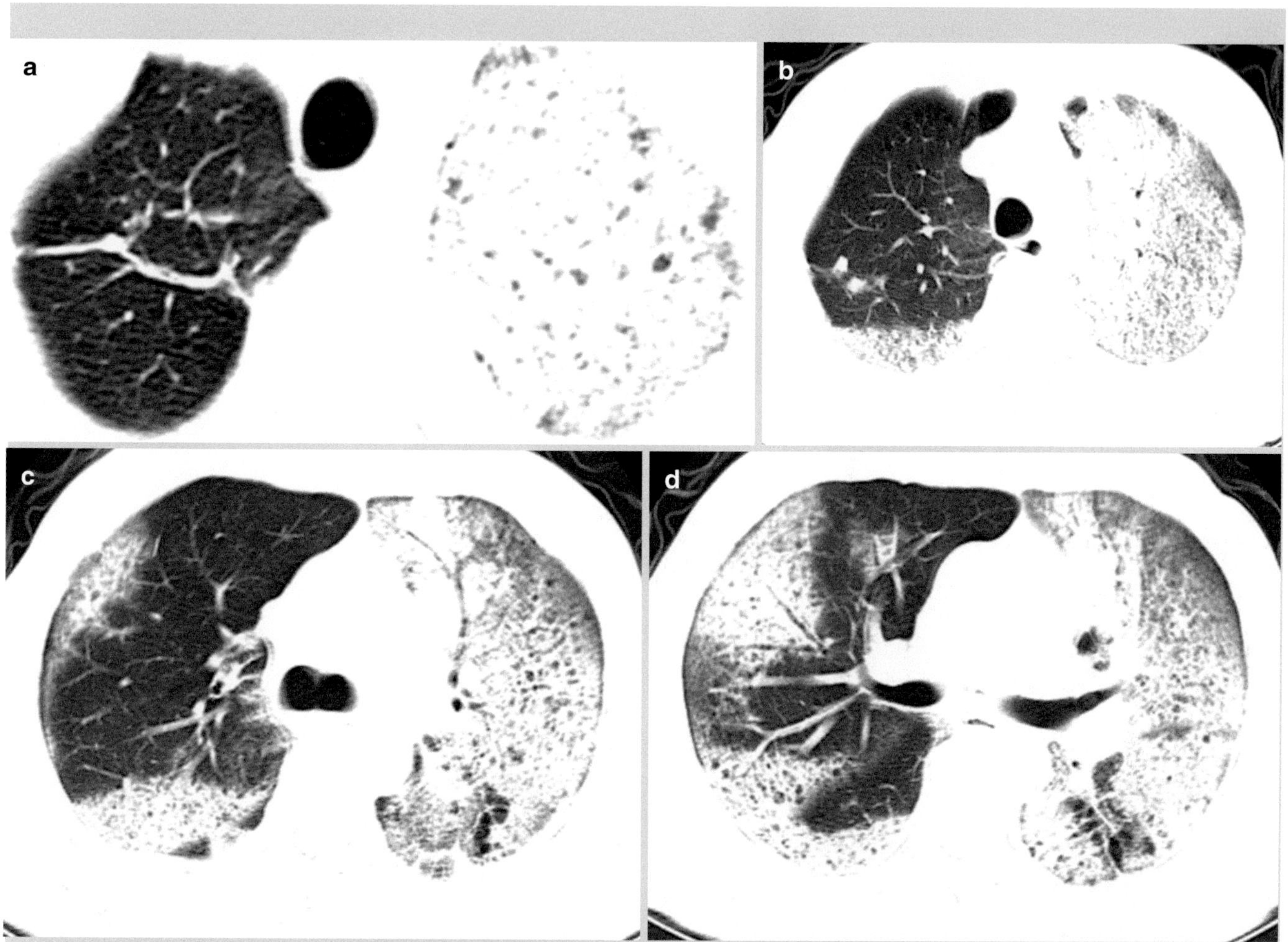

Fig. 12.1 On d 8 after onset, chest CT scan demonstrated large flakes of increased density opacity in the left upper lung; cords like opacity in the right upper lung (**a**). The left upper lung was revealed with large flakes of increased density opacity, with flakes of increased density opacity in the apical posterior segment (**b**). The layer of bronchial bifurcation was revealed with large opacity of increased density in the left upper lung; with strips of increased density opacity in the subpleural area of the right upper lung lobe (**c**). The subcarinal layer was shown with consolidation in the left lung; with flakes of consolidation opacity in the middle and lateral areas of the right upper and middle lung lobes as well as the posterior basilar segment of right lower lung lobe (**d**). The layer of right inferior pulmonary vein was shown with large consolidation in the left lung and the left lower lung; with GGO in the subpleural area of right middle lung lobe and the right lingual lung lobe (**e**). The layer of diaphragmatic dome was revealed with consolidation in the subpleural area of posterior basilar segment of right lower lung lobe and the left lower lung lobe; with lung bullae of 1.5 cm in diameter in the subpleural area of posterior segment of right lower lung lobe (**f**). On d 9 after onset, bedside chest X-ray showed large consolidation in the left lung and the right upper lung field; large GGO in the right middle and lower lung fields (**g**)

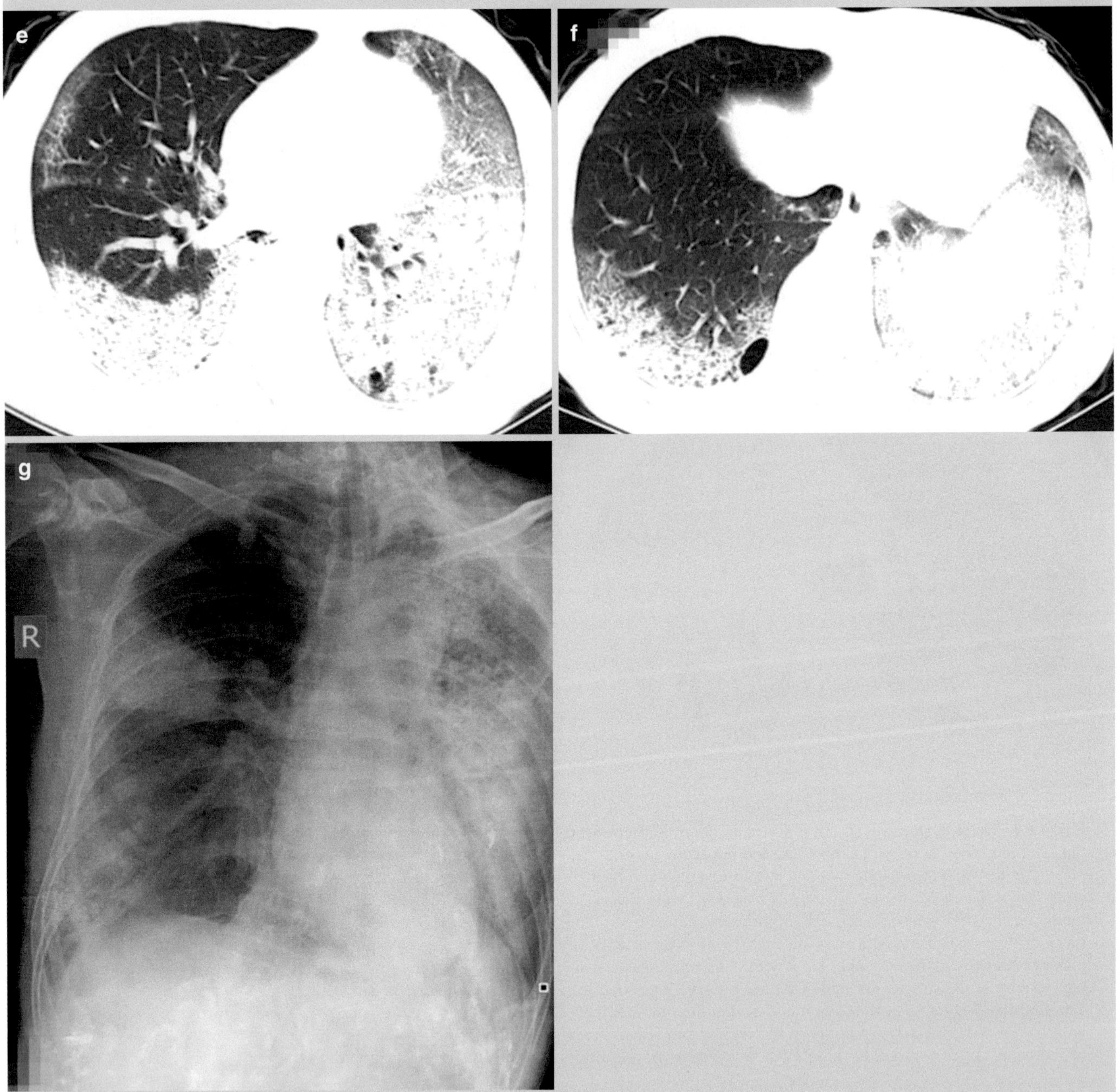

Fig. 12.1 (continued)

Case 2

[Brief Medical History]

A 59-year-old man was hospitalized due to fever for 14 days and shortness of breath for 9 days. Fourteen days prior to his hospitalization, he began to experience fever with his body temperatures fluctuating between 39 and 40 °C and aversion to cold. After oral intake of Compound Pseudoephedrine Hydrochloride tablets by himself, his condition failed to be improved. He experienced no cough, expectoration, hemoptysis, chest distress and pain. Eight days prior to his hospitalization (d 6 after onset), his condition aggravated and he paid his clinic visit in a local hospital. He was preliminarily diagnosed with bacterial infection and given anti-infection therapy (details not known), with poor therapeutic efficacy. Chest X-ray in the local hospital showed multiple infections in both lungs. Routine blood test showed WBC count 6.6×10^9/L, GR% 91.6% and LY% 15.6%; PCT 1.21 ng/ml. Tablets of Ceftazidime and Moxifloxacin Hydrochloride were prescribed to fight against infections, and non-invasive mechanical ventilation was ordered. Six days prior to his hospitalization (d 8 after onset), the patient showed aggravation of shortness of breath, with SPO_2 level of 50–70%. Assisted ventilation via tracheal intubation was then ordered. Meanwhile, throat swab showed nucleic acid of H5 subtype of avian influenza virus positive, fungi positive (++++) in feces, and fungi positive in phlegm, which indicated highly pathogenic human infected avian influenza and severe pneumonia. Medications of Imipenem, Oseltamivir and Ethylprednisolone Sodium Succinate were prescribed, but showing poor therapeutic efficacy. The patient had a medical history of colon cancer 1 year ago, which was treated by sigmoidectomy in another hospital with following 4 sessions of chemotherapy. Reexamination 2 months ago in that hospital indicated no relapse of cancer. More than 30 years ago, the patient had a medical history of pulmonary tuberculosis, which was cured. By physical examination, the body temperature 36.6 °C and SpO_2 95%; assisted ventilation via tracheal intubation; weakened fremitus vocalis by palpation; dullness of both lungs by percussion; weak breathing sounds of both lungs and moist rales of both lower lungs by auscultation. He reported a history of buying a living poultry in a market that provided slaughtering service.

[Radiological demonstration] Fig. 12.2

[Discussion]

In this case of human infected H5N6 avian influenza, poorly defined patches of opacity and consolidation were radiologically revealed, multiple and sporadic, which were exudative lesions. These lesions mainly distributed in the middle and lower lung fields, with both lungs involved, and progressed rapidly, with fusion and extension within a short period of time. And the area with consolidation enlarged to involve multiple lobes and segments of both lungs. These radiological findings are in consistency with literature reports about pneumonia induced by avian influenza virus. On d 14 after onset, CT scan showed pleural effusion in a small quantity, which rarely occurs in the cases of SARS and other avian influenza virus pneumonia. Meanwhile, by deep phlegm culture, acinetobacter baumannii was positive, which may be the reason for pleural effusion. After that, anti-inflammatory treatment was strengthened, and the lesions were gradually controlled and improved.

Radiologically, the disease should be differentiated from bacterial pneumonia, mycoplasma pneumonia and SARS. In the cases of human infected H5N6 avian influenza, the poorly defined patches of opacities distribute in both lungs, with multiple lesions and rapid progression. However, bacterial pneumonia is characterized by limited segmental consolidation and increased WBC count in peripheral blood. Prevalence of mycoplasma pneumonia is seasonal and is more common in children, with lesions in one lung and possibly in both lungs. By radiological follow-ups, the lung lesions in the cases of mycoplasma pneumonia hardly change within a short period of time. And its differential diagnosis from other infectious viral pneumonia is mainly based on epidemiological history and etiological examination.

Fig. 12.2 On d 6 after onset, anterior-posterior and lateral chest X-rays demonstrated multiple poorly defined patches of opacity in both lower lung fields, predominantly in the left lower lung; partial consolidation in the posterior basilar segment of left lower lung; consolidated nodules in the right upper lung (tuberculomas defined by CT scan) (**a**, **b**). On d 8 after onset, reexamination by chest X-ray showed multiple poorly defined patches of opacity and consolidation in the middle and lower lung fields of both lungs, predominantly in both lower lungs; obviously increased lesions (**c**). On d 10 after onset, reexamination by chest X-ray demonstrated multiple poorly defined patches of opacity and consolidation in the middle and lower lung fields of both lungs; poorly defined patches of opacity in the left upper lung field (**d**). On d 14 after onset, chest CT scan showed multiple poorly defined opacity and consolidation in both lungs, predominantly ground glass opacity in the anterior lungs and consolidation in the dorsal lungs; air bronchogram in the consolidation opacity. The lesions predominantly distributed in the dorsal parts of both lower lungs. The lesion of tuberculomas in the posterior segment of right upper lung calcified. Bilateral pleural effusion was shown in a small quantity, more in the left pleural cavity. Partial atelectasis was shown in the posterior basilar segment of both lower lungs due to compression (**e**–**k**). On d 23 after onset, chest CT scan demonstrated obviously decreased lesions in both lungs, relatively decreased pleural effusion and improved atelectasis of dorsal lungs (**l**–**o**). On d 50 after onset, chest CT scan showed absorption of most lesions and sporadic cords like opacity in both lungs (**p**–**s**)

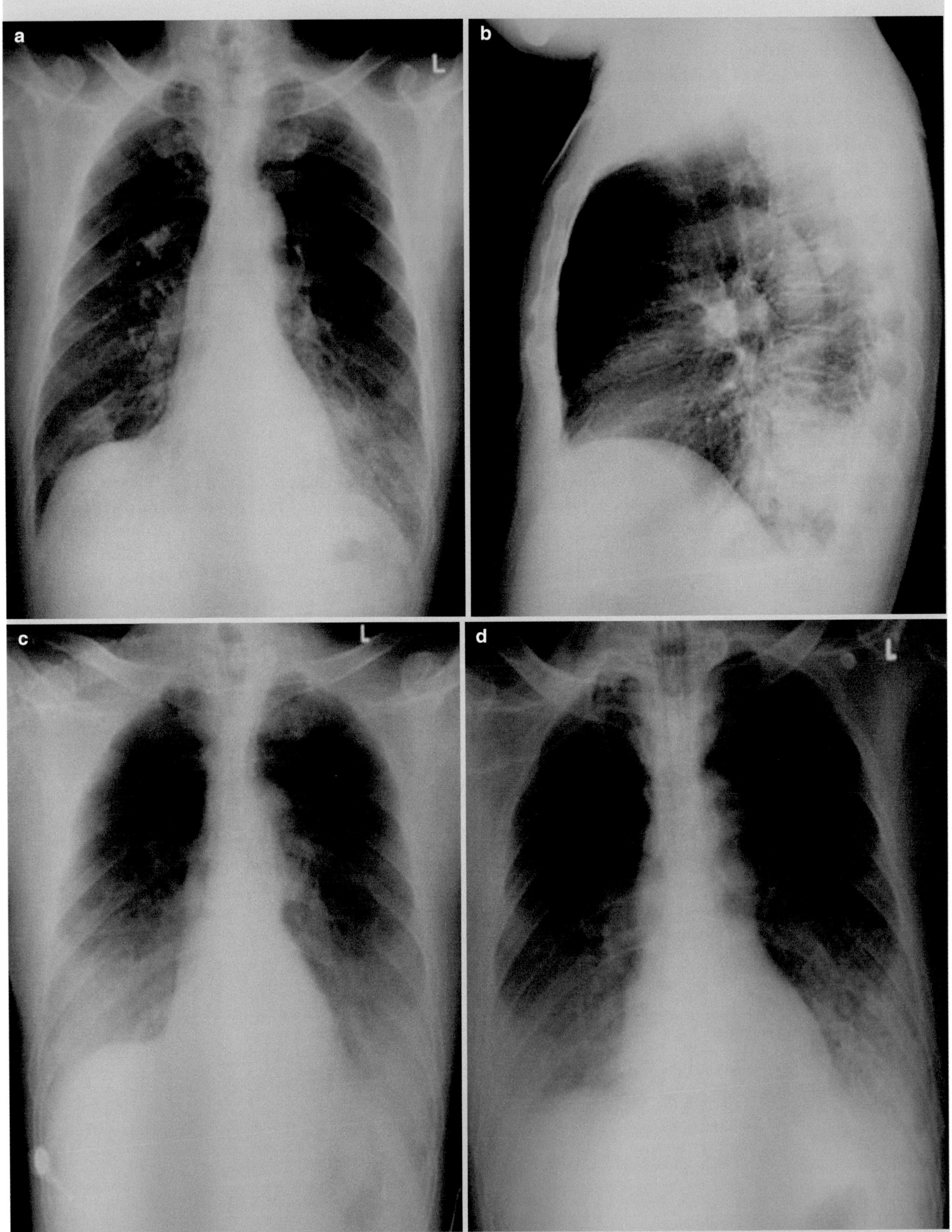

Fig. 12.2 (continued)

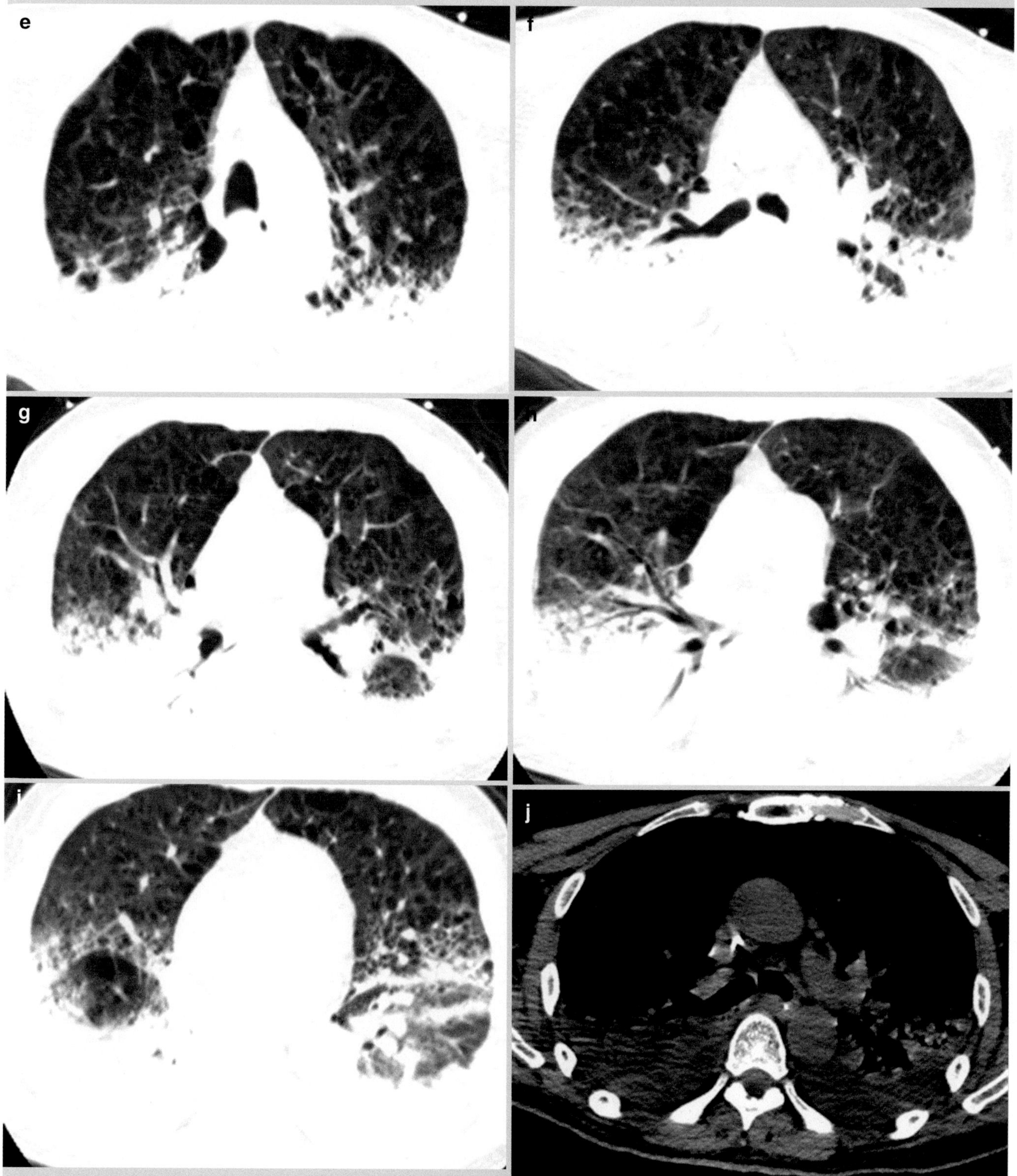

Fig. 12.2 (continued)

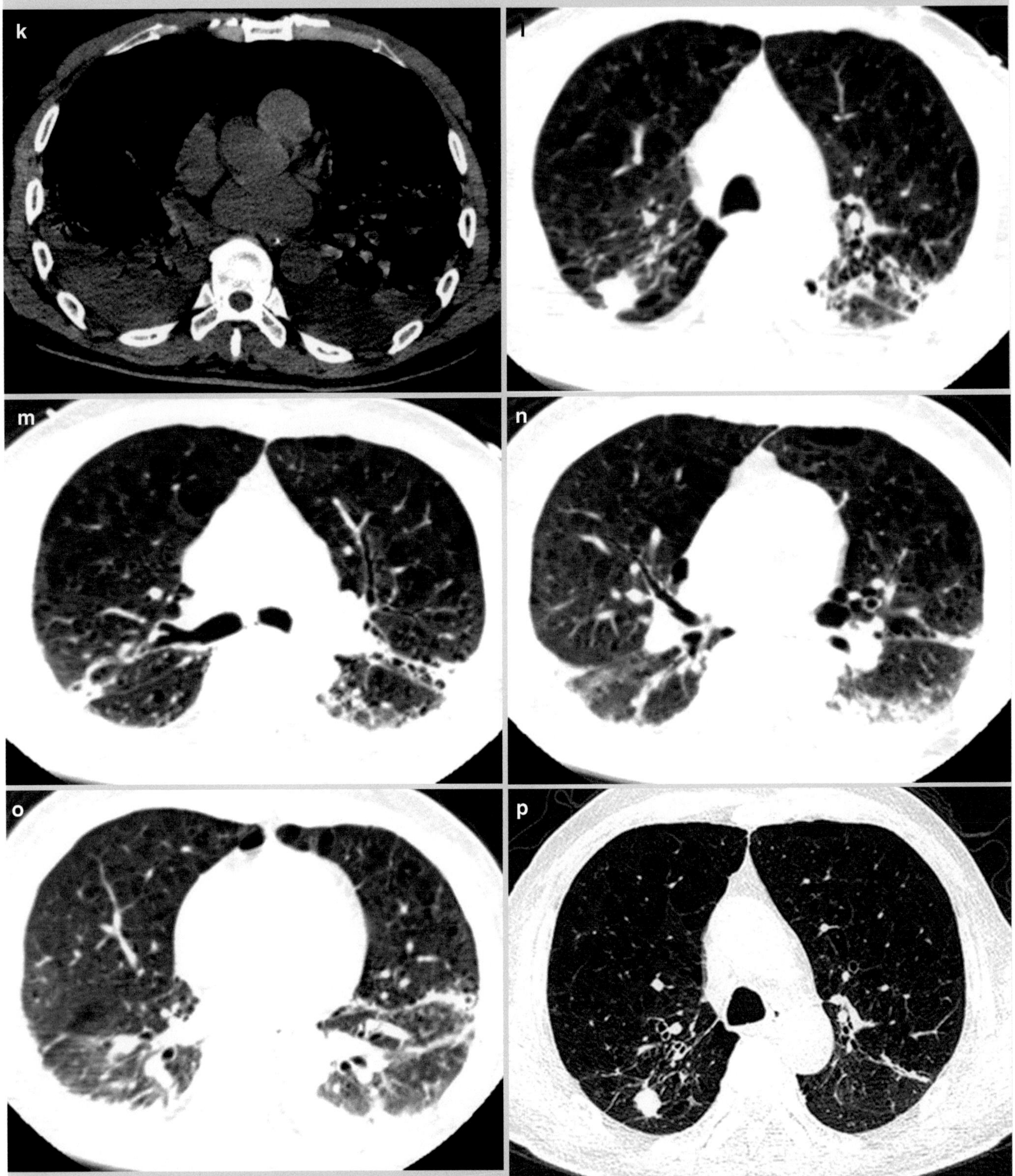

Fig. 12.2 (continued)

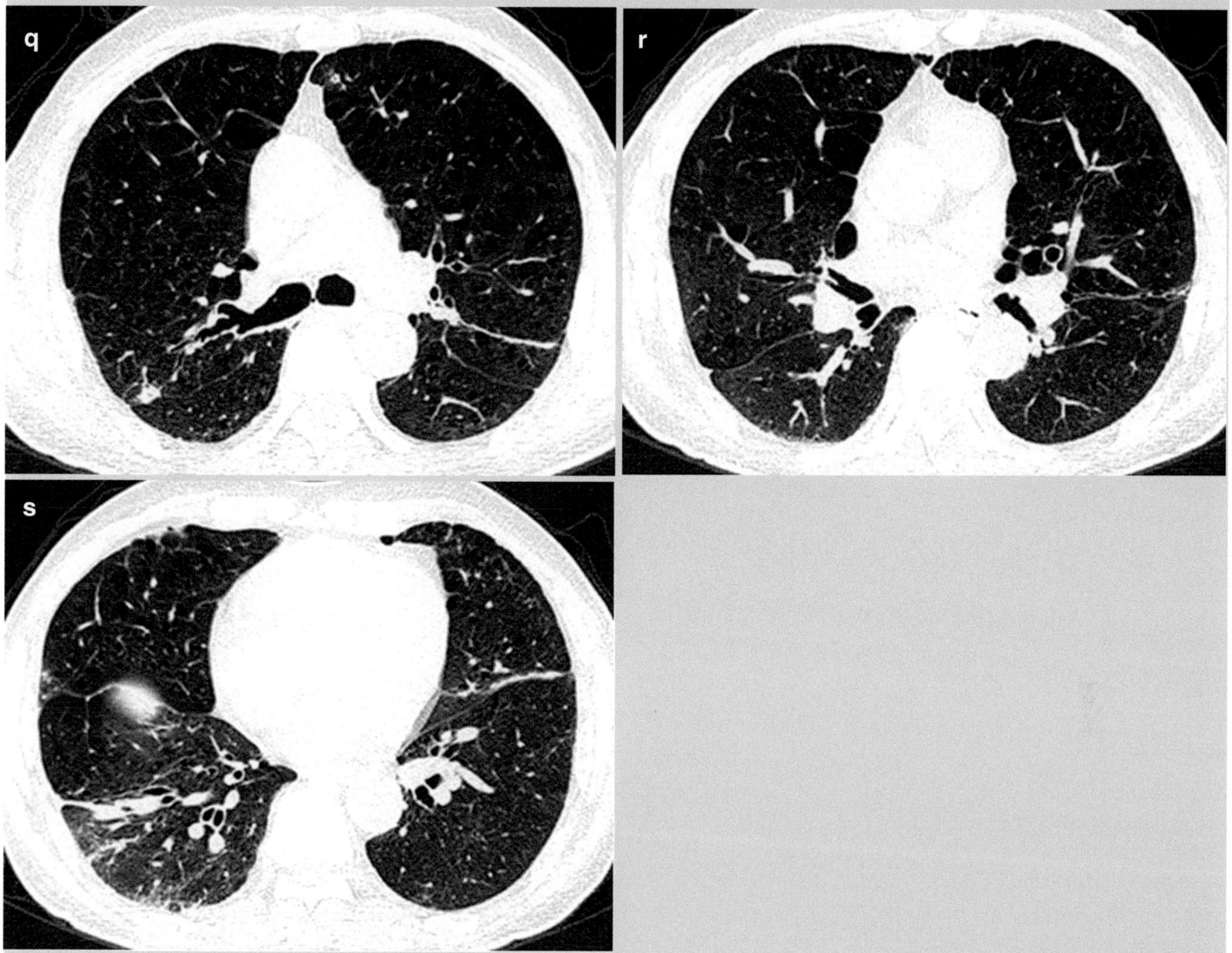

Fig. 12.2 (continued)

References

Lu PX, Zeng Z, Zheng FQ, et al. Radiological demonstrations of severe pneumonia induced by H7N9 avian influenza virus and their dynamic changes. Radiol Pract. 2014;29(7):740–44.

Zeng QS, Chen L, Zhong NS, et al. Diagnosis of SARS by chest X-ray and CT scan. Chin J Radiol. 2003;37(7):600–3.

Zeng Z, Lu PX, Zhou BP. Radiological demonstrations of severe pneumonia induced by H7N9 avian influenza virus. J Tubelcu Lung Health. 2014;3(1):25–8.

Zhou BP, Li YM, Lu PX. Human infected avian influenza. Beijing: Science Press; 2007.

13 Human Infected H10N8 Avian Influenza

Puxuan Lu, Yanan Hu, Jian He, and Xiang Gao

13.1 Introduction

Human infected H10N8 avian influenza is an acute infectious respiratory disease caused by H10N8 subtype of avian influenza virus. On Dec. 6, 2013, 1 death case of severe pneumonia induced by H10N8 avian influenza virus was reported in Nanchang, Jiangxi province of China, which is the first case globally. From Jan. 25 to Feb. 13, 2014, another 2 cases of definitively diagnosed human infected H10N8 avian influenza were successively reported. Death occurred in 2 of the all 3 cases.

H10N8 subtype of avian influenza virus, the same as H5N6 and H5N1 subtypes, is segmental negative-stranded RNA virus and is categorized into the family of Orthomyxoviridae. According to literature report, the first strain of H10N8 avian influenza virus was isolated in specimens from Italian quail in 1965, and a total of 11 strains has been isolated across the world. All these strains were isolated in specimens from poultries, mainly wild birds. In the year of 1995, De Marco MA, an Italian scientist, successfully isolated H10N8 avian influenza virus from serum of chicken. It has ever been reported in China that 2 strains of avian influenza virus were isolated, one in water samples from Dongting Lake wetland by Wuhan Institute of Virology in 2007, one in ducks from a market selling living poultries by Provincial Institute of Zoology of Guangdong, China in 2012. To study the pathogenicity of H10N8 avian influenza virus in mammals, researchers in Wuhan Institute of Virology conducted experiments on mice and chickens, revealing no virus in venous blood and nose of chickens. And thus they reported that H10N8 avian influenza virus is mildly pathogenic to chickens. However, the experiments showed that the virus replicates in mice lungs, their virulence correspondingly increases that is strong enough to cause death, and the virus is detectable in tissues of various organs and brain.

P. Lu (✉)
Affiliated Shenzhen Third People's Hospital, Guangdong Medical College, Shenzhen, Guangdong, China
e-mail: lupuxuan@126.com

Y. Hu
Guangzhou University of Chinese Medicine, Guangzhou, Guangdong, China

J. He • X. Gao
Nanchang First People's Hospital, Nanchang, Jiangxi, China

After human is infected with H10N8 avian influenza virus, the condition rapidly deteriorates, with a high mortality. However, direct sources of its infection remain unknown and the effective measures for its prevention and treatment are insufficient. Therefore, it is necessary to molecularly study the pathomechanism of avian influenza virus across the species barriers to infect mammals and humans, and to molecularly study the essential conditions of gene mutations and recombinations that enable avian influenza virus to infect human respiratory tracts and replicate there. The questions about limited person-to-person spread of H10N8 avian influenza virus and possibility of its pandemics after gene mutations or recombinations still remain to be studied in detail.

13.2 Typical Cases

Case 1

[Brief Medical History]

A 73-year-old woman experienced cough, expectoration, chest distress after physical activities and shortness of breath since Nov. 27, 2013. But she experienced no fever, stomachache, diarrhea, urinary frequency and urgency. Onset of fever with accompanying aversion to cold occurred at night on Nov. 29, 2013 and she was hospitalized on the following day. The patient had medical histories of high blood pressure and coronary heart disease. In Dec 2012, she suffered from myasthemia gravis and thymoma, which was treated by thymectomy. Medication of pyridostigmine after operation, 60 mmHg 3 times per day helped to control her condition. By physical examination, the body temperature was 39.1 °C, breathing rate 32/min and blood pressure 116/80 mmHg. She was well conscious, with shortness of breath but no cyanosis. By auscultation, coarse breathing sounds in both lungs and fine moist rales in the right lung but no wheezing. The heart rate 98/min, sinus rhythm; abdomen negative and muscle strength normal. On Dec. 6, 2013, death occurred due to respiratory failure and shock.

H. Li (ed.), *Radiology of Influenza*, DOI 10.1007/978-94-024-0908-6_13

The patient reported that she had no history of visiting other places 2 weeks before onset, no history of contact to patients with fever and influenza like symptoms, no family visitors and no influenza like symptoms in her family members. On Nov. 23, 2013, she, together with the part-time household maid, ever bought a living chicken in an agricultural market 1000 m away from her home. The stall keeper picked one chicken for them, which was then preliminarily processed at the stall. The patient stayed there for about 5 min and then left. At home, the part-time household maid processed the chicken and cooked it for chicken soup, during which the patient did not enter the kitchen. At that time, only the maid and the patient were at home. After cooking, the knives and chopping block were cleaned immediately and the knives were separately used for the raw and cooked food at home. After thymectomy, the patient never ate chicken and drank chicken soup, and the chicken soup was for the dinner of her son, daughter-in-law and granddaughter at that night. According to investigation, 17 persons were confirmed to have close contact with the patient, and all of them received medical observation, showing no clinical manifestations of fever and respiratory symptoms. The medical staff with close contact to the patient received throat swab test, showing negative to common primer of type A influenza virus.

Routine blood test on Nov. 30, 2013 showed WBC count $10.34 \times 10^9/L$, N 0.764, L 0.070, PLT $124 \times 10^9/L$, and CRP>200 mg/L. Blood glass analysis revealed pH 7.48, PO_2 57 mmHg, and PCO_2 32 mmHg. On Dec. 1, 2013, laboratory test showed CK 10KU/L, myoglobin 62 μg/l, and LDH 187 U/L. Kidney function test showed Creatinine 35.7 μg/l. Liver function test on Dec. 4 revealed ALT 25 U/L, AST 57 U/L, and ChE 1978 U/L. Electrolytes test revealed K^+ 4.2 mmol/L, Na^+ 120.2 mmol/L, and Cl^- 88.8 mmol/L.

On Dec. 5, 2013, the test performed by the National Central Laboratory of Influenza in China revealed the nucleic acid of H10N8 avian influenza virus positive, and the strain was officially nominated as A/Jiangxi-Donghu/346/2013(JD-H10N8), abbreviated as JX346. By sequencing and comparative analysis, the virus is derived from avian influenza virus and its internal gene is from H9N2 avian influenza virus. The sputum test, blood culture, and viral nucleic acid test failed to detect bacterial infection, fungal infection and infection of other subtypes of avian influenza virus.

[**Radiological demonstration**] Fig. 13.1

[**Diagnosis**] Pneumonia induced by human infected H10N8 avian influenza virus.

[**Discussion**]

It has been speculated that H10N8 subtype of virus may firstly infect wild birds to induce H10N8 avian influenza virus, followed by its infection of poultries. It is likely that recombination of H10N8 AIV genes with H9N2 AIV genes in infected poultries produces a new strain of H10N8 avian influenza virus containing internal genes of H9N2 AIV.. Six internal genes of JX346 (H10N8) strain are from H9N2 AIV, whose biological properties resemble to H5N1 and H7N9 subtypes of AIV. In addition, H10N8 and H7N9 subtypes of avian influenza virus share the commonalities of weak pathogenicity in wild birds and poultries, but increased pathogenecity after their infections of human, which indicated that avian influenza virus of weak pathogenecity dramatically changes after it crosses species barriers. As far as we know, H5N1, H7N9, H6N5 and H10N8 subtypes of avian influenza virus can infect human and cause death. It should be paid attention that 6 internal genes of H5N1, H7N9 and H10N8 subtypes of avian influenza virus are from H9N2 subtype of avian influenza virus, indicates these internal genes from H9N2 subtype may facilitate to enhance their pathogenicity to human and may be closely related to their changes of virulence. The receptor binding site of JX346 (H10N8) HA protein contains 226–228 amino acid residues, namely QSG, indicating JX346 (H10N8) possesses properties of AIV and is more likely to bind with the receptor of α2, 3Gal-SA, while common influenza virus is more likely to bind with the receptor of α2, 6Gal-SA and JX346 (H10N8) may be capable of binding with the two receptors. The receptor of α2, 6Gal-SA mainly distributes on the surface of upper respiratory epithelia while the receptor of α2, 3Gal-SA in lower respiratory tract, which may be partially responsible for the lower respiratory infection in this case of H10N8 subtype avian influenza virus infection that caused severe pneumonia.

This is the globally first case of human infected H10N8 avian influenza, with an incubation period of about 4 days, which is close to the incubation period of human infected H5N1 or H7N9 subtype of avian influenza. The early clinical symptoms of human infected H10N8 avian influenza include fever, cough, and chest distress. Laboratory blood test may show decreased lymphocytes, increased neutrophils and WBC count, elevated C-reactive protein and creatinine concentration, and decreased blood IgG and complement C3.

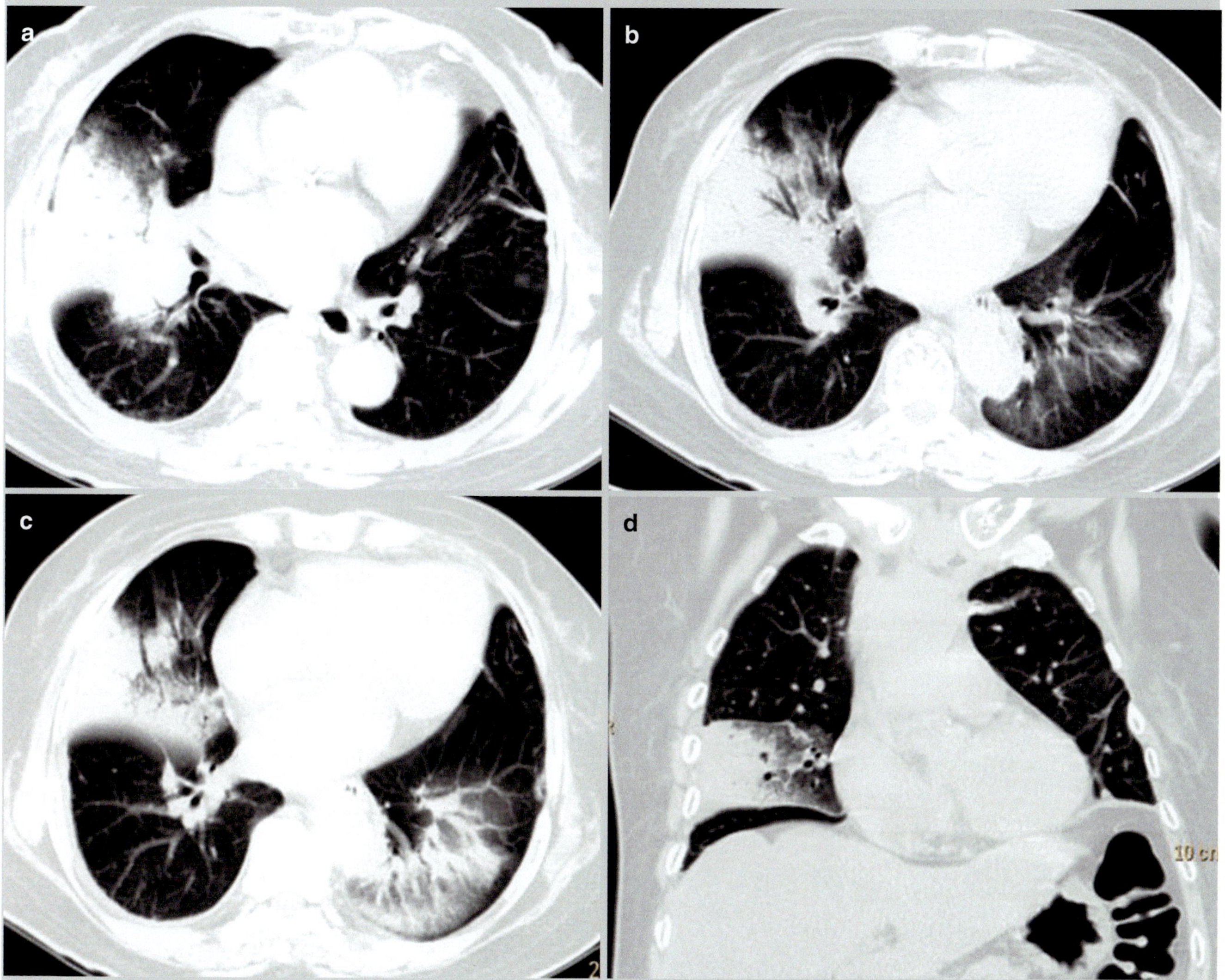

Fig. 13.1 On d 4 after onset, chest CT scan demonstrated large consolidation opacity in the right middle and lower lung lobes; patches of consolidation and ground glass opacity in the left lower lung lobe (**a**–**d**). On d 6 after onset, bedside chest X-ray showed obvious progression of the large consolidation and ground glass opacities in both lungs; and enlarged blurry hilum opacity in both lungs (**e**). On d 7 after onset, bedside chest X-ray showed increased lesions in both lungs (**f**). On d 8 after onset, bedside X-ray demonstrated white-lung sign of both lungs (**g**)

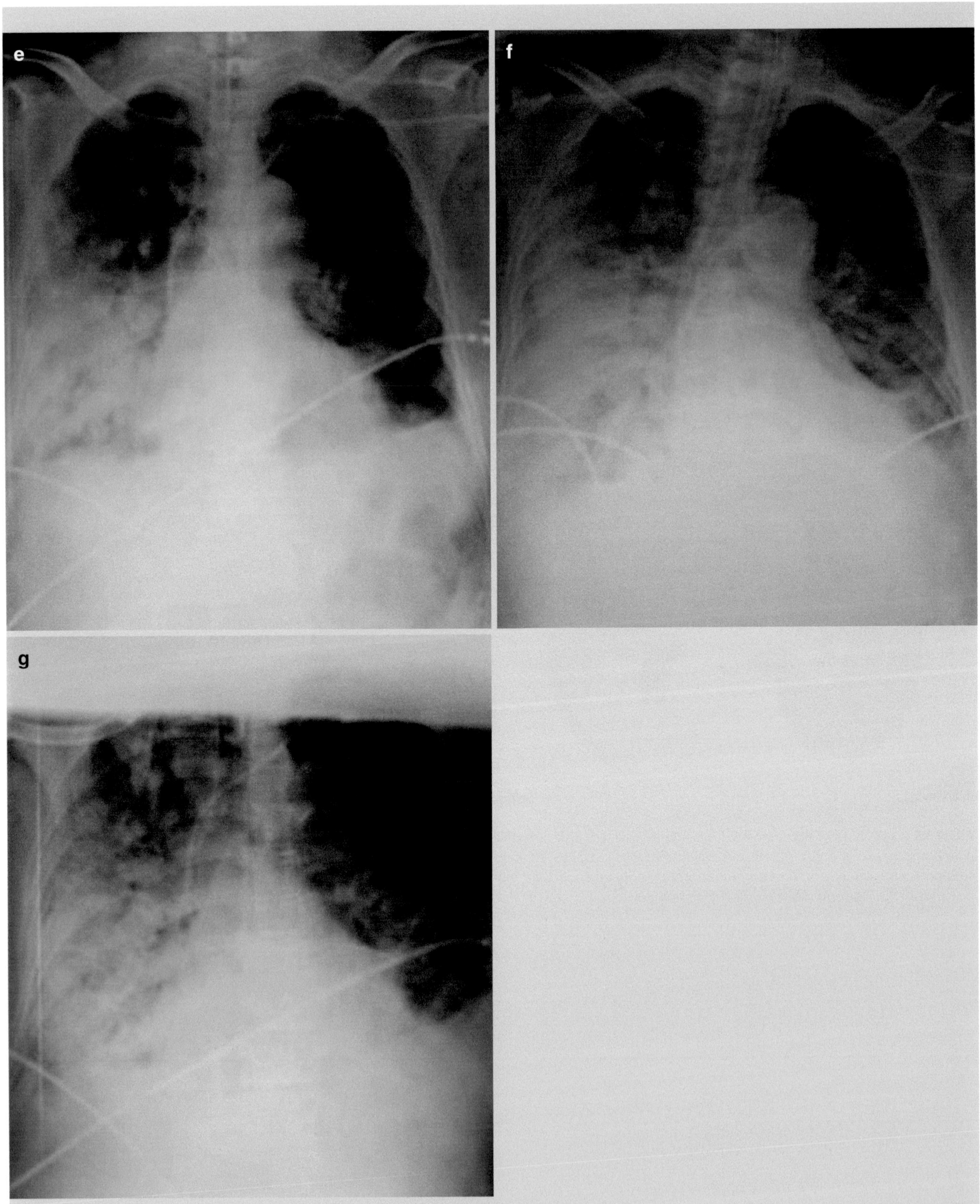

Fig. 13.1 (continued)

Even though anti-viral, anti-bacterial and hormone therapies were given, the condition of the patient rapidly deteriorated in the late stage, with occurrences of severe pneumonia, septic shock, acute renal failure and multiple organs dysfunction. Death occurred on d 6 after hospitalization. Although the patient reported a history of exposure to a market selling living poultries, no H10N8 subtype of avian influenza virus was detected in environment monitoring samples and no influenza like symptoms showed in persons who had a history of close contact to the patient after medical observation for 2 weeks. And their antibodies tests targeting on the H10N8 subtype of avian influenza virus showed negative, indicating H10N8 subtype of avian influenza virus is incapable of person-to-person spread. The sputum test, blood test and viral nucleic acid test of the patient showed negative to bacterial infection, fungal infection and the other subtypes AIV infection.

Concerning radiological examination, chest CT scan on d 4 after onset demonstrated patches and large flakes of opacity with increased density in the right middle and lower lung and the left lower lung field, predominantly consolidation opacity; obvious air bronchogram in the consolidations of the right middle lung lobe; flakes of GGO in the left lower lung. The lesions mainly distributed in the middle and lower lobes of both lungs, with their shape and density predominantly as large flakes of consolidations. Bedside chest X-ray on d 6 after onset showed rapid progression of the lesions in both lungs, with enlarged consolidation opacity in bilateral middle and lower lung fields, large GGO in the right upper lung and the left middle lung field, and enlarged poorly defined hilum opacity in both lungs. Meanwhile, physical examination showed low blood pressure of 72/40 mmHg, heart rate 160/min, oxygen saturation 72 %, and pinkish foamy sputum in the endotracheal intubated canula, indicating possibilities of heart failure and pulmonary edema. The radiological findings were in consistency with the clinical manifestations. Chest X-ray on d 7 and d 8 after onset showed further progressed lesions in white-lung sign of both lungs. The lesions are radiologically characterized by the followings:

The lesions mainly onset in bilateral middle and lower lung fields, early as large consolidation opacity in both lungs with rapid progression. During the progressive stage, the lesions are mainly consolidations and GGOs, with observable pleural effusion in a small quantity. Radiologically, it should be differentiated from pneumonia induced by other subtypes of influenza A virus. In terms of onset location, shape and density of the lesions, it resembles to pneumonia induced by H7N9 avian influenza virus, and their differential diagnosis should be mainly based on epidemiological history and etiological examination. During its early stage, it should also be differentiated from bacterial pneumonia. The patients with bacterial pneumonia experience fever, cough as well as increased WBC count and neutrophils. By CT scan, bacterial pneumonia is demonstrated as consolidation opacity in lung lobes and segments. However, pneumonia induced by human infected avian influenza virus is demonstrated as extensive lung lesions with rapid progression as well as concurrent consolidation and GGO.

References

Chen HY, Yuan H, Gao RB, et al. Clinical and epidemiological characteristics of a fatal case of avian influenza A H10N8 virus infection: a descriptive study. Lancet. 2014;383(9918):714–21.

Fu WJ, Hu MH, Liu XQ, et al. Retrospective analysis of severe pneumonia induced by H10N8 avian influenza virus: report of 1 case in Jiangxi province of China. Chinese Journal of Public Health. 2014;30(6):818–9.

Wan JG, Zhang JX, Tao WQ, et al. Analysis of the globally first case of severe pneumonia induced by H10N8 avian influenza virus. Chinese Journal of Critical Care Medicine. 2014;26(2):120–2.